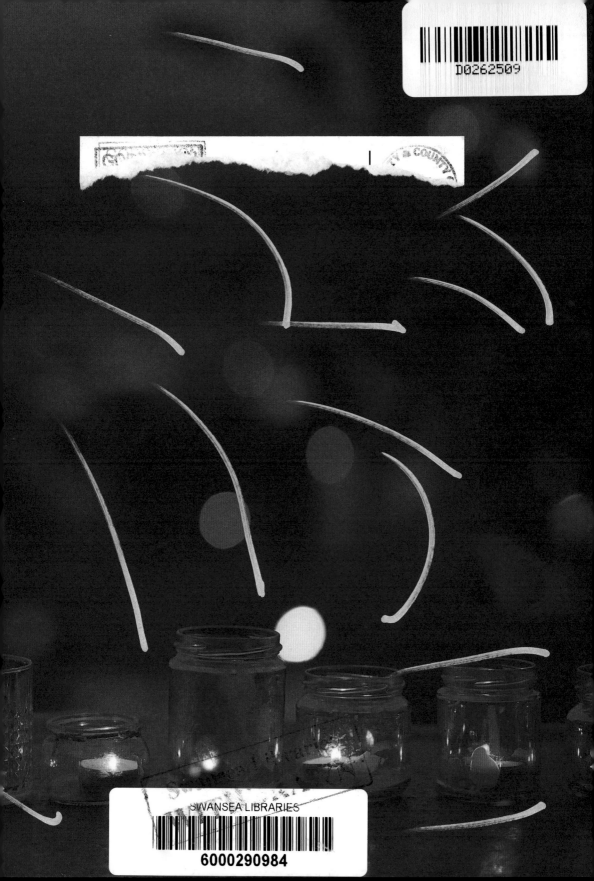
D0262509

SWANSEA LIBRARIES

6000290984

Deliciously
Ella with
Friends

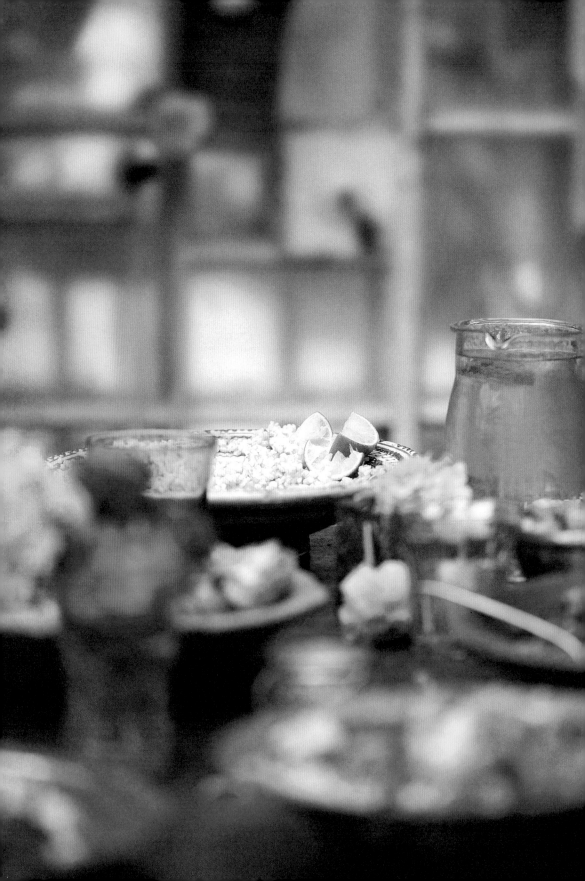

Deliciously
Ella with
Friends

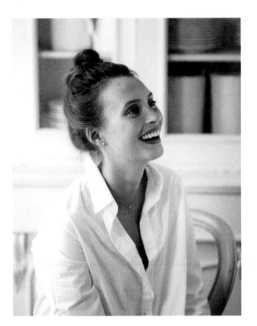

yellow
kite

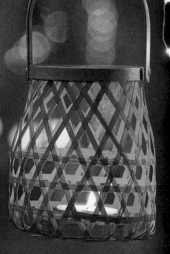

*This book, like everything I do, is for my readers.
Thank you for giving me the opportunity to share
health and happiness with you every day. Your love
of my recipes inspires me more than I can say.*

*It's also for my husband Matthew and our amazing
team at Deliciously Ella and the MaE Deli; without
their love and support, none of this would be possible.*

CONTENTS

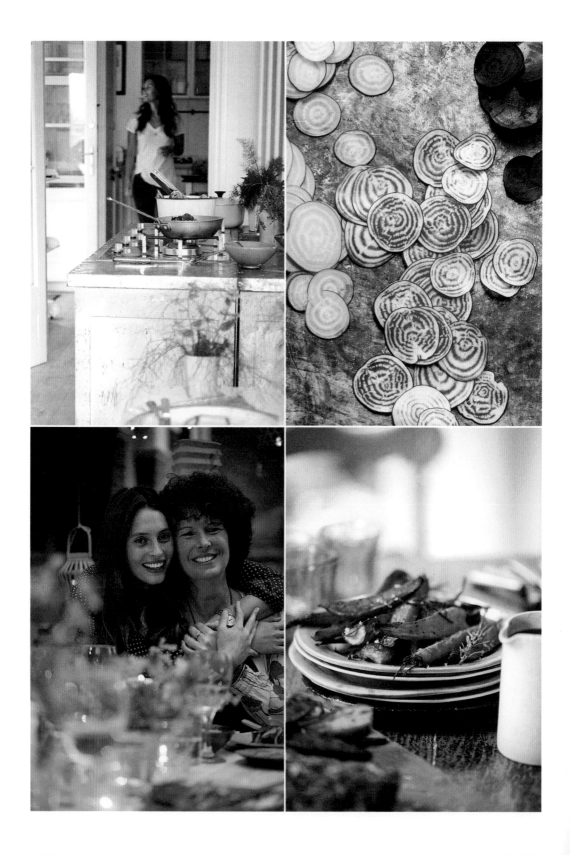

INTRODUCTION

Over the last few years healthy eating has really grown in popularity, which has been wonderful to watch! It's given me such a thrill to see people realise how good they feel when they eat foods that nourish their bodies. The best part of it all, though, is that everyone's started to see how incredibly delicious healthy living can be. The stereotype that it's all about lettuce and cucumber is vanishing and is being replaced with dreamy visions of blueberry pancake stacks with caramelised banana bites and crunchy cacao and almond butter, bowls of creamy sweet potato noodles with satay sauce, mango and mushroom ceviche and chocolate orange tart.

So many of my readers say that they love eating wholefoods and incorporating plant-based meals into their routine… but that their husbands, wives, children, friends and colleagues are more sceptical and, as a result, they're not particularly open-minded about trying new, veggie-laden dishes. Lots of people also struggle to know what to cook and how to put menus together when they're entertaining, especially when they're new to this way of eating. When I first started eating a plant-based diet, I found it hard to know which dishes would complement each other best. I got it really wrong a few times with my friends and I'm pretty sure they left the table thinking I was a bit mad! The good news is that this book is designed to solve both these issues.

Each chapter is focused on delicious meals. I've got your mornings covered with brunches and breakfasts; followed by lighter meals that work well on the go; big healthy feasts and celebration menus; essential side dishes; party staples; and, of course, everyone's favourite - desserts. I've also given meal suggestions that cater to your every sociable need: think brunch for the girls, or a grab and go breakfast, storecupboard saviours, delights for your desk, cold weather comforters, Mexican fiestas and even dishes – such as a knockout

Sunday lunch – designed to impress the sceptics in your life! So once you've worked your way through the book you'll feel inspired, knowing exactly how to put Deliciously Ella-style meals together in a way that persuades your friends and family to try some healthy versions of their favourites. Plus, you'll get to cook more than 100 delicious new recipes. We'll be making so many lovely things, from peanut butter and jelly cake to quesadillas stuffed with garlicky beans, cashew sour cream, salsa and guacamole; almond butter rocky roads; pea, courgette and coconut risotto; chickpea chilli with baked sweet potatoes; and chocolate peanut butter pie! Get ready: this is a seriously tasty book.

We'll start with my favourite breakfast and brunch recipes: think on-the-go menus with crumbly blueberry squares, roasted almond butter bars and honey and lemon breakfast bars. Or awesome savoury brunches with stacks of sweet potato rosti piled high with maple and rosemary butter beans and spread with a thick layer of herby guacamole. We're also having toasted buckwheat and coconut granola with zesty mango and pineapple bowls and passion fruit yogurt, as well as baked garlicky tomatoes, scrambled turmeric and red pepper tofu and thyme fried mushrooms. There's a great range of options, from easy dishes you can throw together to help rushed mornings when you're time poor, to fancy brunches to share on lazy weekends.

We'll then go through some fantastic lighter recipes that work well for quick weekday suppers, as well as portable lunches. We'll look at fresh bites like mango and mushroom ceviche and sushi rolls filled with cauliflower rice, sesame and avocado; after-work catch-up menus of spiced potato cakes with garlicky tomato sauce and green beans; and perfect picnics with charred coconut corn and vibrant salads filled with mango, pepper, cucumber and a peanut dressing. This chapter is full of my go-to meals, quick and easy, but still so delicious!

The chilli and ginger pho, sesame slaw, pistachio and apricot quinoa and sesame and maple summer rolls are real favourites here. I make these for Matt and I during the week when we're at home, or when I have a couple of girlfriends coming over for weekday supper.

The next chapter is all about hearty feasts and celebrations, these are the meals I make when I have lots of friends and family over, or want to impress someone! I promise all these dishes and menus will convince any sceptic that eating well can be pretty amazing. There's a great selection of ideas in here, from Mexican-themed feasts, to curries with home-made lime pickle, to warming meals of tomato and aubergine bake served alongside bowls of spinach with mustard seeds. We then cover everything from garden parties filled with charred cauliflower steaks on a bed of chilli quinoa and sun-dried tomato and butter bean hummus, to comforting bowls of three bean stew with mango salsa, to simple, inexpensive suppers of spiced chickpea chilli stuffed into baked sweet potatoes. There's really something for everyone.

After this we move towards side dishes. This is probably my favourite chapter of the book as there's such a wide range of ingredients, flavours and textures here. I absolutely love using these as traditional sides, but it's also fun to make a few of these recipes and throw them into a bowl together to make a full meal, it always looks beautiful and tastes sensational. I have so many much-loved recipes in this chapter, but the baked plantains with a sweet chilli sauce, the smashed potatoes with turmeric and mustard seeds, the miso and sesame glazed aubergines and the spicy baked avocado fries with their lime, cashew and coriander dip are all absolute winners... and you all should try them, I have a feeling that they'll become staples in your diet too. There's a good mix of impressive and simple dishes in this chapter, so there should be something to suit every taste bud and every occasion. The other great thing about the recipes in this chapter is that you can mix and match them with just about anything, so if you're not ready to go fully Deliciously Ella, then just add these to your existing go-to meals. That way you can experiment with new ingredients without it all feeling too new and overwhelming. If you're a meat eater, then these are great ways to incorporate a bit more plant-based goodness into your diet too, and hopefully they'll get you excited about how good veggies can taste.

To make things more fun I've dedicated a whole chapter to parties; we've got nibbles, cocktails and mocktails and even birthday teas! You'll be able to serve a lovely array of little bites, from charred Padrón peppers with chipotle cream to bowls of smoky baked tortilla chips with babaganoush, aubergine rolls with a minty coconut tzatziki and mini baked potatoes with cashew sour cream and chives, as well as mini socca pizza bites. To accompany them there's a list of mocktails and cocktails, so you and your friends can sip

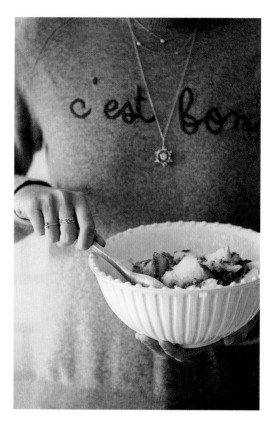

on sparkling pineapple and cayenne drinks, or watermelon and cucumber coolers as you catch up. And to end the chapter we've got a beautiful afternoon tea with iced ginger muffins, a banana and raisin cake and simple cucumber and lemon butter bean hummus open sandwiches, as well as a birthday tea with peanut butter and honey flapjacks, blueberry scones with vanilla coconut cream and a triple-layered celebration cake. I think this chapter will really show your friends and family that healthy eating is accessible, delicious and sociable – it's absolutely not about sitting on your own at home every night meditating and eating kale salad! These dishes are amazing if you want to do a big dinner party, too, as they mean you can keep it delicious but with a healthy twist from start to finish!

To end the book we'll go through all the best sweet ways to finish a meal. I know how much my readers love sweets and there are some real winners in this chapter, which I'm sure you'll all really enjoying making, eating and sharing (if there's any left by the time your friends arrive!). We've got beautiful desserts like pistachio and orange truffles, watermelon and mint granita, pan-fried cardamom and honey apples and berries with creamy chocolate sauce and crushed nuts, which work so well as lighter options at the end of a meal. There are also lots of amazing snacks, from salted maca and tahini fudge, to orange and cardamom cookies and my personal favourite – quinoa, hazelnut and cacao bars – that work really well on the go. Then, if you're looking for something heartier and more indulgent there are some wonders for you towards the end of the chapter as we move towards chocolate peanut butter pie, glazed orange polenta cake and even a sticky toffee pudding. There's so much here for everyone, and I'm sure these will all go down really well with your friends and family.

Hopefully the recipes, ideas and menus that you'll see throughout the book will inspire you to get cooking, so that you can enjoy amazing food with the people you love. Of course, you don't have to use the book in this way; I pull out single recipes and make them on their own all the time, as they're all so great and obviously you won't necessarily want to make a full three-course meal every night! I've just put them together to help you work out what goes well with what, so that you feel confident in the kitchen.

HOW TO MAKE HEALTHY EATING APPROACHABLE FOR EVERYONE

While I am on the subject of sharing food with others, including those who might be more sceptical about eating plant-based food, the other point I'd like to highlight is that eating well is not about labels, guilt or enforcing a certain way of eating on yourself or anyone else. It's so important to remember this, especially when you're introducing your friends and family to this kind of food, as you don't want them to feel too overwhelmed and daunted by the concept.

The way we eat is so personal to us, and we are all different. We have different bodies, different medical histories, different genes, different lifestyles and different tastes. I do believe that everyone is better off – both physically and mentally – with a diet full of fruit, veg, nuts, seeds, beans, legumes, healthy grains, and less refined sugar and processed food… but, after that, you have to make your own decisions, and it's OK if these are different to the choices made by your friends and family. Only you know what's practical, enjoyable and sustainable for your lifestyle and, as with anything in life, the way you eat doesn't fall into a one-size-fits-all bucket.

Healthy eating is about finding a way of eating that makes you happy. It's about meals that make you feel your best – that might mean a crumbly blueberry square for breakfast, a lemony potato and butter bean salad for lunch… and then a pizza with wine for dinner with friends - and that's totally OK. It's your body and your life. Yes, I want to encourage everyone to show their bodies some love and take good care of them, but I never ever want anyone to feel guilty because they're not eating 'perfectly' all the time. Plus, there is no such thing as perfect – perfect is simply finding a balance that is right for you, whatever that is.

This book is all about natural, plant-based food and the recipes are all vegetarian and wheat-free, but there are no labels on any of it, it's simply about delicious food that's designed to help you feel good, and you can adapt any of it. As you read this book, please don't feel you have to put yourself firmly into any dietary 'category'. Putting yourself in a certain box with a specific label can be quite restrictive. You just shouldn't feel that you're not healthy if you're not specifically raw, plant-based, paleo, grain-free, gluten-free, wheat-free or any of the rest of it. You can absolutely be a bit of everything, you just have to be honest with yourself and work out what makes you feel best… and that might be a happy mix of everything. Of course it can also mean following a certain concept, but please don't feel as though it's wrong if you don't. Likewise, you shouldn't expect anyone else you know and love to categorise themselves either. Don't forget that healthy eating should never be prescriptive or restricting!

The other thing to note is that we also all want to commit to healthy eating to different extents and that's great. I eat the way I do because I love it, but also because it's also the only way that I'm able to manage my illness. I want to – and have to – eat nourishing food all the time. Just because I eat this way every day, though, doesn't mean you should feel bad if you don't. Similarly, you shouldn't inflict guilt on anyone else if they're not ready to eat healthily all day long either, just focus on encouraging them to add more natural foods to their diet and celebrate the small steps and changes that they're making rather than focusing on the other things you feel they could be doing. We all respond so much better to positivity than negativity.

So please remember that when you're introducing friends and family to this food, it's important to let them know that it's totally OK to be a flexible healthy eater and that – just because you live with someone or spend a lot of time together – it doesn't mean you have to eat in exactly the same way. Everyone has to start somewhere, at some point, and it's much better to introduce healthy living to your own or someone else's life in a sustainable way over time than it is to do it all at once… and then quit three days later because you/ they hate living off kale salads.

Find a balance that works for you and the people around you, incorporate whole ingredients and nourishing foods whenever you can and – most importantly – please don't beat yourself up or make anyone else feel bad for eating something that isn't super-healthy… because life is much too short for that!

MY OWN EXPERIENCE

When I first starting eating this way, about five years ago, my friends and family thought I was mad. They supported me with my diet change as I was so ill and they were willing to be enthusiastic about anything that I thought would help, but they had no idea what I would eat and they all thought it would be a pretty depressing culinary experience! I'm happy to say that I proved them wrong though: they all began to love it quite quickly and now these foods play a big part in their lives, too. As I suggested earlier, I won them round by simply adding Deliciously Ella side dishes to our meals; this meant that they were still enjoying familiar dishes as the main part of their plates, which then made them more open-minded to trying something else as an extra, as it felt less strange and intimidating. After a while they started to ask for my dishes, without me even suggesting them and, now, without me even being there.

I felt a bit lonely when I started out enjoying all these lovely foods on my own, so it was a real joy when my friends and family started loving them too. I really think there's something very special about creating beautiful dishes for the people you love and enjoying them together. I've seen this both at home with my friends and family, but also at work, as Deliciously Ella has expanded into supper clubs and the MaE Deli.

One of the reasons I think my supper clubs have been so popular is that people feel it's such a great way to introduce the food they love to the people they love, so lots of them bring colleagues, partners and friends. I always host the clubs in warm, welcoming spaces and have big menus filled with a great mix of dishes that aim to cover everyone's wants and needs. I make an effort to include familiar items, like stews with brown rice and brownies, and find that all the guys go straight to those! I've seen the same success with familiar food at the MaE Deli too. We created a menu where you can choose to have a bowl of sweet potato falafel, veggie quinoa, charred broccoli and spiced hummus... but you can also bring a more sceptical friend and they could enjoy a big bowl of brown rice with Thai curry and a side of organic chicken. I'm constantly amazed at how well this way of introducing people to healthier options works. I love seeing how it can bring people together too: it's really lovely to see a person who – like me – can't eat lots of things, be able to pick anything off the menu and then share it with someone who matters to them.

I really hope that you can get your friends and family on board too and all share in the same deliciousness soon!

TOP TIPS FOR ENCOURAGING FRIENDS AND FAMILY TO GET HEALTHIER

1 FOCUS ON FAMILIAR FOOD

If you're having a real sceptic for dinner, or trying to get an unconvinced family member to try a healthier meal, then always cook something that looks and feels familiar to them. Choose a classic dish with a healthy spin on it. Something like the Indian feast in this book with bowls of coconut rice, chana masala and aloo gobi. This is a perfect meal, as your guests are never going to look at it and think, 'What is that, it looks terrifyingly healthy!' and decide they don't like it before they try it, plus it's really satisfying and hearty, which means everyone will go home full. So remember to go easy on everyone, don't leap straight to raw food, or anything too unfamiliar and scary looking!

2 DEMONSTRATE, DON'T PREACH

No one likes to be preached at or made to feel guilty about anything in life, especially the way they eat, as it's often attached to a lot of emotions and possibly deep-rooted insecurities. Don't talk about meals as being 'good' or 'bad' health wise: there's no point categorising anything to inflict guilt. Instead just demonstrate how delicious healthy food is. Make your friends amazing, nourishing meals and encourage them to try them, but without telling them why it's so much better than what they normally eat. Simply cook and share natural goodness; that's exactly how I got all my friends and family involved. If you do want to inspire them with the benefits of healthy eating, then let them know how good you've been feeling since you started incorporating more wholefoods into your diet, and how much your own energy levels – and everything else – have improved... but just don't go on about it too much!

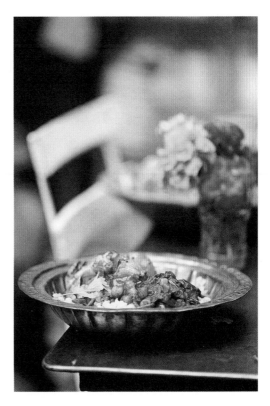

3 IT'S OK TO ADAPT ALL THE RECIPES

As I said earlier, healthy eating isn't about labelling yourself or forcing yourself to do something you don't enjoy. If you're new to healthy eating, or trying to get friends and family involved, don't be afraid to adapt any of my recipes to make them more accessible for your audience. If adding chicken, fish, cheese or eggs makes the people you love more likely to try something new, then add them in by all means; if it makes them more receptive and allows them to enjoy the meal more, then that's a great thing. It also means their plate will look more familiar, which I find is the best approach.

4 DON'T CHANGE EVERYTHING AT ONCE

You don't have to overhaul your diet overnight. There's no rush or deadline for changing your lifestyle, it's about finding an enjoyable, sustainable way of life that makes you happy and it really doesn't matter how long it takes to get there! Start by focusing on positives and adding goodness in, rather than taking everything away. Add in new veggie dishes throughout the week, but don't feel you have to remove the old favourites at the same time; just let the two coexist for a while as you get used to new ways of eating and cooking. Allow yourself and the people around you however long you and they need to start loving the new ingredients, textures and tastes. Most importantly, never criticise yourself if you don't enjoy something! You don't have to love all fruit and veg, even I don't enjoy them all – you'll never find me eating Iceberg lettuce or green peppers for example – but that's OK, there are so many other lovely ingredients out there to experiment with instead.

5 DON'T BE TOO STRICT ON YOURSELF OR ANYONE ELSE

It's so important to remember that no one is perfect, and there's no point in striving for perfection, as the concept simply doesn't exist. This is relevant to everything in life really, but

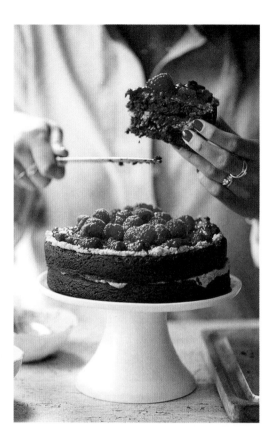

I believe it's especially important to remember when thinking about food. When it comes to what we eat and how we eat, we just have to do what makes us feel happiest and never forget that this will be different for everyone. Food is such an important part of life and you don't want to feel stressed every time you sit down for a meal, that takes away all the fun from something you should really look forward to and savour. So find a balance that you enjoy and, if you lapse from your healthy-eating plan, never beat yourself up, just find a positive way to get back into it; we're all only human after all! Every change in life also takes time to become a habit, so don't expect yourself to wake up craving quinoa on day one; sadly it's unlikely to happen. Just be OK with that, accept where you are right now and, crucially, don't judge what you are craving: embrace it… and then try to incorporate a healthy something on the side!

6 MAKE THE MEAL BEAUTIFUL

Concentrate on making the food you serve look really appetising. It may sound like a bit of a waste of time, but it's not. We eat with our eyes first, so a dish needs to look tempting, especially if you're trying to get someone new excited about it. If you and your guests think it looks amazing you'll all be much more open-minded and ready for it to taste amazing, too. This has been one of the most important things for me as Deliciously Ella, especially on the blog and Instagram. So many readers have said that they tried something they thought they wouldn't like because it looked great, and they ended up loving it! It doesn't take long to enhance the appearance of something, you just need to put it in a clean, beautiful serving dish (rather than serving it in what you cooked it in) and then add a little colour and texture with dressings, herb sprinklings and toppings such as toasted nuts and pomegranates.

7 KEEP THE INGREDIENTS A SECRET

This may sound a bit strange, but I find it really helps people be more objective if they don't know there's a certain ingredient in a dish. Lots of us think we hate a particular taste or texture but, if we try it in a new context, we often end up loving it. I've had so many friends say 'Oh I hate dates,' but then they love my crunchy almond butter rocky roads and eat three of them, or they say they hate coriander but adore the spiced potato cakes. Especially if it's just one of many ingredients, it's worth keeping it a secret so that they try it with an open mind... and I think you'll both be surprised by the result! (Obviously, make sure you know they are not allergic to it first.) If it is a main ingredient, and therefore not disguisable, then I always highlight the fact that it's been cooked in a totally different way and is being served with new flavours, to demonstrate that it's very different to how they may have had it before, and this often works too. Just do your best to encourage your friends and family to try things with an open mind and you may end up with a few new converts!

I hope my experiences, and the tips I've learned for convincing friends and family to try new things, are helpful to you all. Now, let's get cooking!

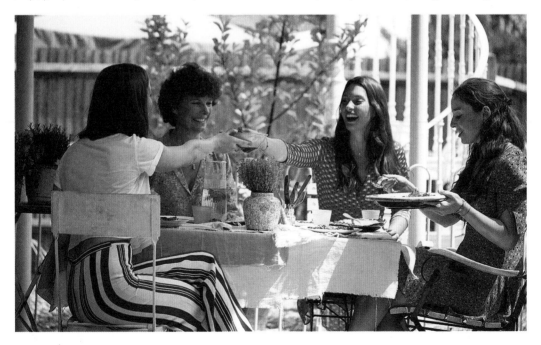

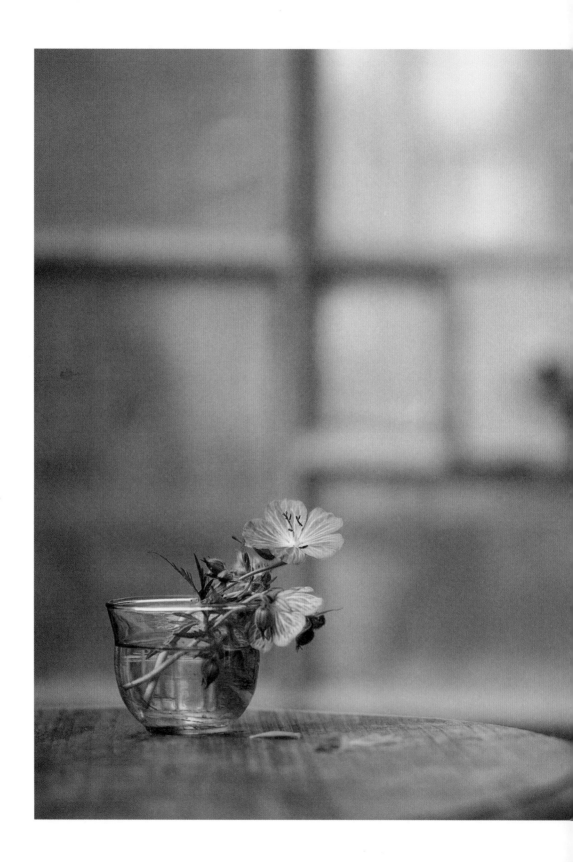

MORNINGS

BREAKFASTS & BRUNCHES TO MAKE EVERY DAY DELICIOUS

MORNINGS

I'm a big breakfast person. I really believe that it's the most important meal of the day, and it tends to be the one I'm most excited about. Some days I'm really busy so I'll grab a Honey & Lemon Breakfast Bar and a Crumbly Blueberry Square to eat on the go as I run out of the door. Other days I have time to throw together a Zesty Mango & Pineapple Bowl with Passion Fruit Yogurt and a sprinkling of Toasted Buckwheat & Coconut Granola for Matt and myself, and we can spend a few minutes savouring the flavours before the day starts. On weekends I like to invite friends over for long, leisurely brunches and really take my time over the meal, so you'll find me feasting on a Blueberry Pancake Stack with Caramelised Banana Bites and dollops of home-made Crunchy Cacao & Almond Butter.

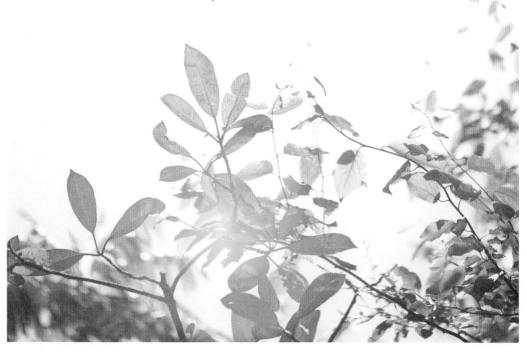

MENUS

GRAB & GO
Honey & Lemon Breakfast Bars
Crumbly Blueberry Squares
Roasted Almond Butter Bars

US TIME
Matt's Berry & Orange Smoothie
Toasted Buckwheat & Coconut Granola
Zesty Mango & Pineapple Bowls with Passion Fruit Yogurt

SWEET BRUNCH
Blueberry Pancake Stack
Caramelised Banana Bites
Crunchy Cacao & Almond Butter

THE NEW FULL ENGLISH
Scrambled Turmeric & Red Pepper Tofu
Thyme Fried Mushrooms
Garlicky Baked Tomatoes

SAVOURY BRUNCH
Sweet Potato Rosti
Maple & Rosemary Butter Beans
Herby Guacamole

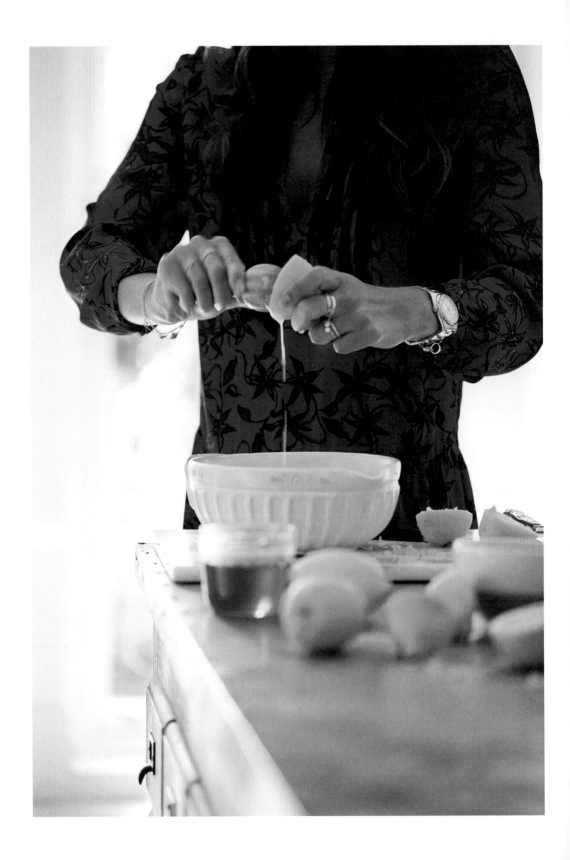

HONEY & LEMON BREAKFAST BARS

These are easy to carry around, full of flavour and simple to make. They also freeze very well, so you can make a big batch and they'll last you a long time. If you like a sweet snack in the afternoon, too, take an extra bar with you to enjoy later in the day.

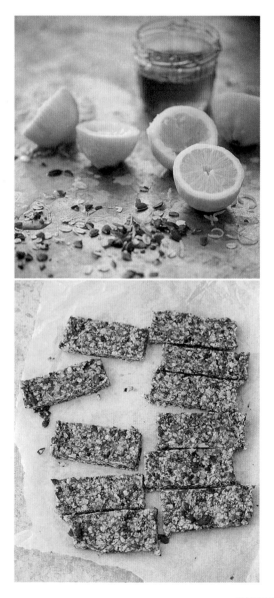

Makes 8

NUT-FREE

1 tablespoon coconut oil
3 tablespoons runny honey
juice and finely grated zest of 1 unwaxed
    lemon
1 tablespoon tahini
70g pumpkin seeds
6 medjool dates, pitted
110g oats
2 tablespoons chia seeds
pinch of salt

Melt the coconut oil, honey, lemon juice and tahini together in a pan over a gentle heat.

Put the pumpkin seeds into a food processor and pulse a few times until they are roughly chopped. Tip into a large mixing bowl. Put the dates in the food processor and blend until a sticky paste forms. Add this to the pumpkin seeds with all the other ingredients, including the contents of the pan (and not forgetting the lemon zest). Mix thoroughly until everything is evenly coated.

Line a baking tray or large lunch box with baking parchment, spoon in the mixture and press it down evenly.

Place in the fridge for about 2 hours to set. Cut into squares or slices before serving.

CRUMBLY BLUEBERRY SQUARES

I make a big batch of these every week or two, so I have great speedy options to grab when I'm running out of the house to start the day. That makes my mornings so much simpler... and way more delicious.

Makes 16

NUT-FREE

FOR THE BASE

a little coconut oil, for the tin

375g oats

100ml brown rice milk, or other
    plant-based milk

5 tablespoons maple syrup

½ teaspoon ground cinnamon

FOR THE FILLING

300g blueberries

2 tablespoons maple syrup

6 medjool dates, pitted and
    roughly chopped

2 teaspoons ground arrowroot

FOR THE TOPPING

4 tablespoons coconut oil

2 tablespoons honey

1 teaspoon ground cinnamon

½ teaspoon ground ginger

200g jumbo oats

Preheat the oven to 180°C (fan 160°C). Use the coconut oil to oil a 20cm square brownie tin.

Start by making the base. Place all the ingredients into a food processor and pulse-blend a few times, until everything is mixed but not totally smooth. Press the mixture into the prepared tin, packing it as tightly as you can. Pop it in the oven for 15 minutes, then take out and set aside to cool.

Next make the filling. Simply place all the ingredients except the arrowroot into a saucepan with 50ml of water and place over a medium heat for about 10 minutes until the blueberries have all burst and it's starting to resemble a compote. Stir in the arrowroot and 2 more teaspoons of water to help it thicken. Set aside to cool.

Meanwhile, make the topping. Melt the coconut oil, honey and spices together in a saucepan, then stir in the oats.

Pour the berry filling on to the base and spread it out evenly, then tumble over the oaty topping, pressing down lightly so that it is compact and completely covers the filling. Return it to the oven for 25–30 minutes, until the top is golden. Leave to cool in the tin before cutting into portions.

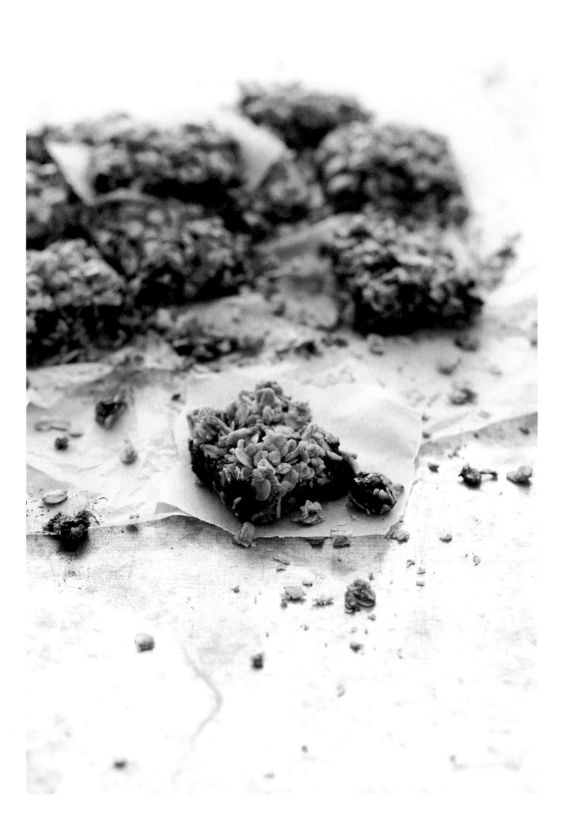

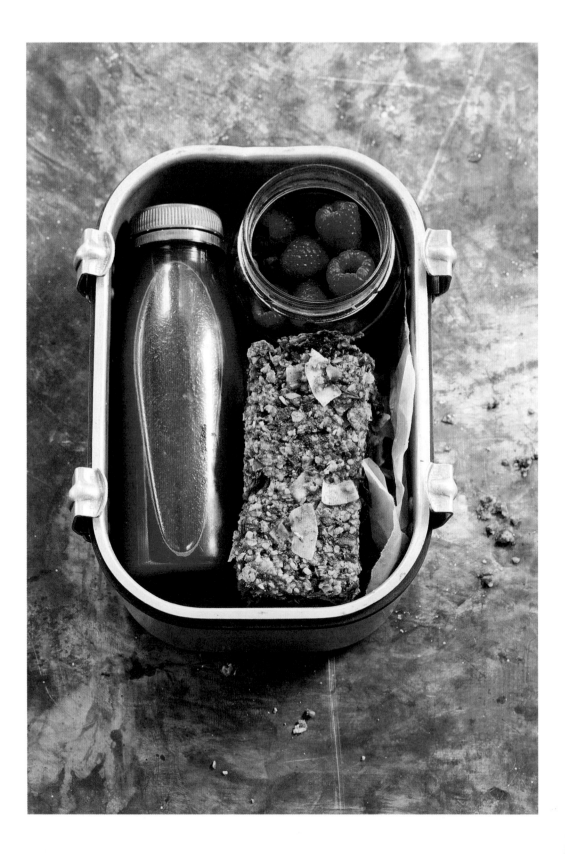

ROASTED ALMOND BUTTER BARS

An ideal option for busy mornings, wonderfully chewy with little bites of juicy raisins, coconut chips and hemp seeds. I use dates and apple purée to sweeten these, so they're not overly sweet and sickly, making them a great way to start your day!

Makes 10–12

2 tablespoons coconut oil, plus more
   for the tin
2 tablespoons chia seeds
12 medjool dates, pitted
200g oats
5 tablespoons Apple Purée (see below)
2 teaspoons ground cinnamon
4 tablespoons hulled hemp seeds
3 tablespoons roasted almond butter
30g coconut chips
60g raisins
pinch of salt

Preheat the oven to 200°C (fan 180°C). Use coconut oil to oil a 26 x 18cm baking tin.

Put the chia in a glass with 8 tablespoons of water. Let this sit for 20 minutes until the seeds expand and form a gel.

Put the dates and the 2 tablespoons of coconut oil into a food processor and whizz.

Mix all the other ingredients, including the chia gel, in a bowl, then stir in the dates until everything is evenly blended.

Press into the prepared tin and bake for about 20 minutes, or until golden brown.

CLEVER COOKING

Apple purée is a great way to sweeten lots of recipes without adding refined sugar. Simply peel and core red apples and chop them into bite-sized pieces. Place in a large saucepan with 2cm of water. Simmer for 40 minutes, or until very soft, then blend until smooth. Store in the fridge for up to 5 days, or freeze in portions.

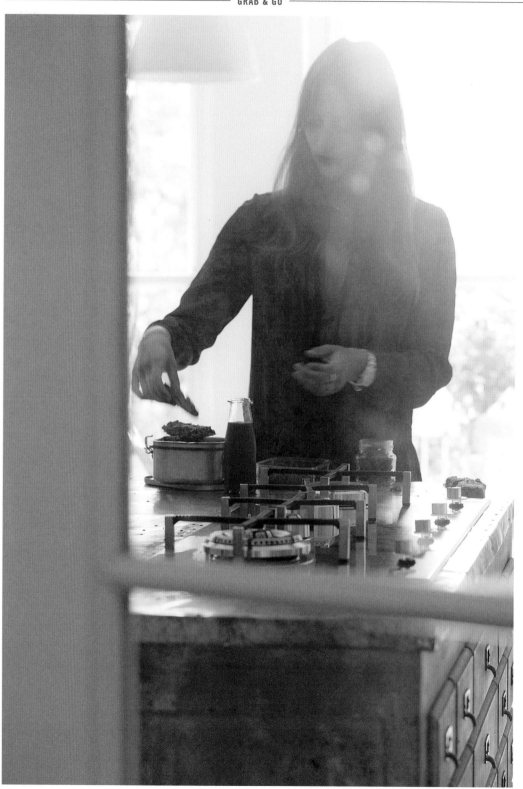

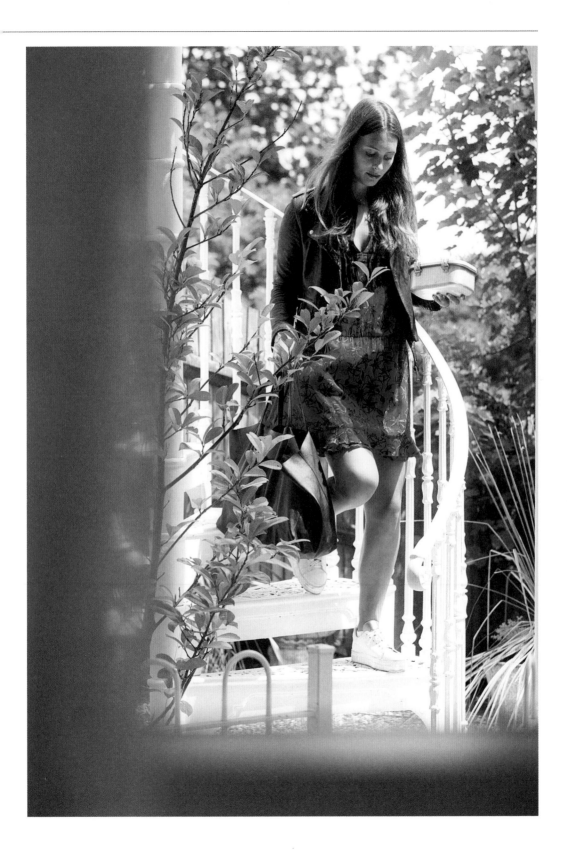

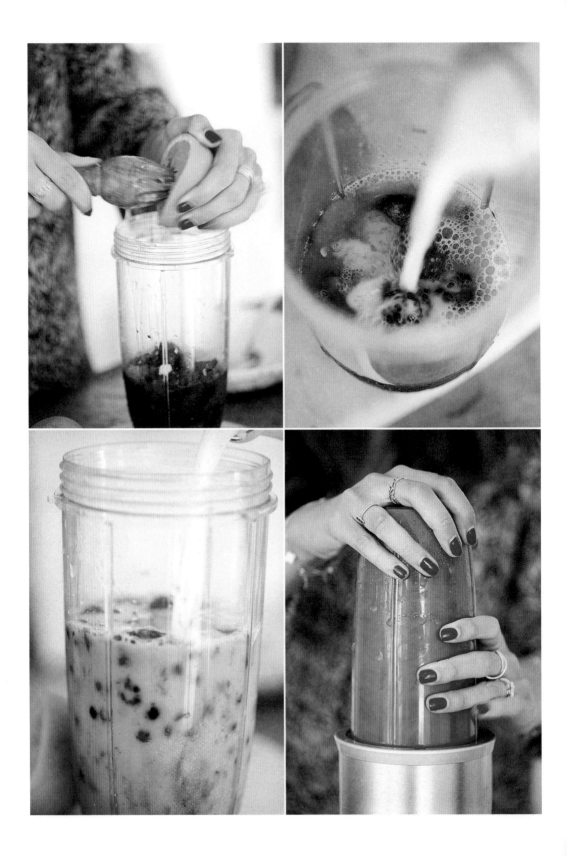

MATT'S BERRY & ORANGE SMOOTHIE

I've made this smoothie for Matt pretty much every morning for the last year! He's totally obsessed with it, and luckily for me it's easy to throw together. The frozen berries give it a lovely thick texture, while the orange and honey add great sweetness to every sip. It's a great accompaniment to Zesty Mango & Pineapple Bowls sprinkled with crunchy granola (pages 30 and 29).

Makes 1 large glass

NUT-FREE

2 oranges

150g frozen mixed berries

100ml brown rice milk, or other
   plant-based milk

½ teaspoon honey (optional)

Cut the oranges in half and use a citrus squeezer to juice them into a blender.

Tip all the other ingredients into the blender, and blend until smooth.

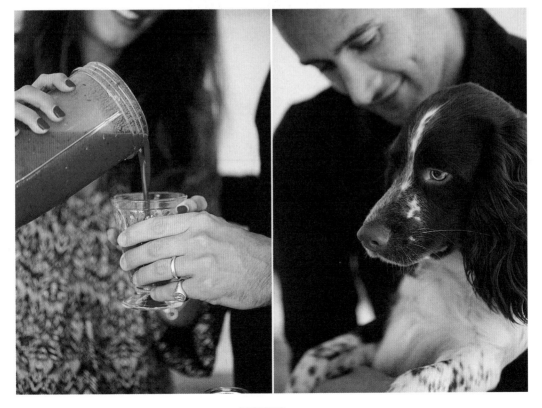

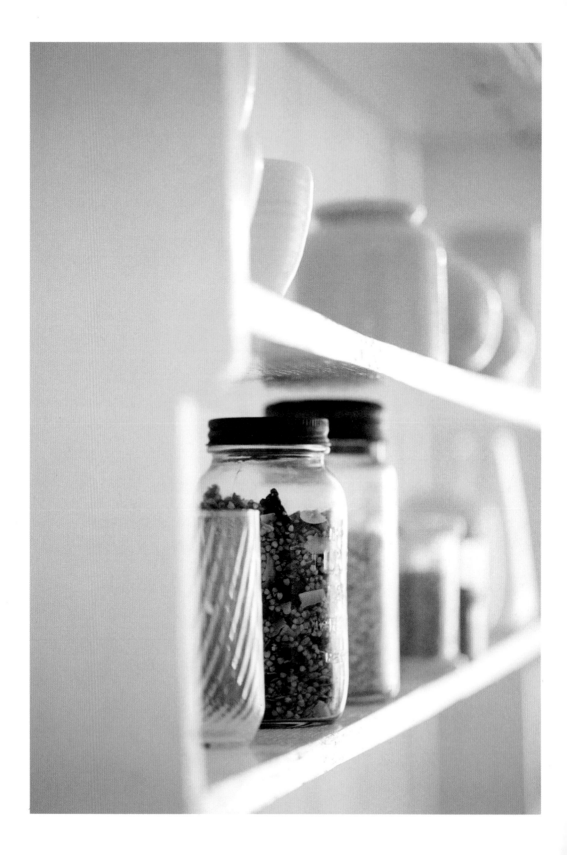

TOASTED BUCKWHEAT & COCONUT GRANOLA

I'm a complete granola addict, it's one of my favourite breakfasts, snacks and sweet treats. For me the best thing about munching on a handful of granola is the crunchy texture, which is just so incredibly satisfying. Using buckwheat groats instead of oats makes each bite especially crunchy, which is why I love this recipe so much. I toss the buckwheat in coconut oil, honey, ginger, cinnamon and vanilla, then bake it all together until my kitchen smells divine and my tummy starts rumbling!

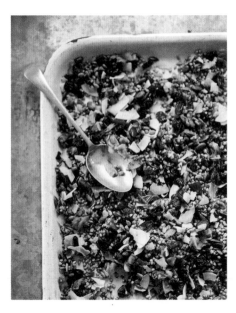

Makes 1 jar

NUT-FREE

300g buckwheat groats

60g coconut chips

50g sunflower seeds

100g pumpkin seeds

pinch of salt

3 tablespoons coconut oil

3 teaspoons ground cinnamon

5 teaspoons ground ginger

2 teaspoons vanilla powder

3 tablespoons honey

40–60g dried cranberries, preferably
   unsweetened (optional)

20–40g raisins (optional)

Preheat the oven to 200°C (fan 180°C).

Mix the buckwheat, coconut chips and seeds in a bowl with the pinch of salt.

Warm the coconut oil, cinnamon, ginger, vanilla and honey in a pan, heating gently until everything is mixed and the coconut oil has melted. Pour into the buckwheat bowl and mix everything together. Spread out evenly on a baking tray.

Bake for 15 minutes, then give it a good stir.

Bake for another 10 minutes, stirring it halfway through.

Let it cool, then, once at room temperature, stir in any dried fruit you want and store in an airtight container. It will last in there for a couple of weeks.

ZESTY MANGO & PINEAPPLE BOWLS
WITH PASSION FRUIT YOGURT

*The sweet passion fruit yogurt here tastes amazing with the mix of mango, pineapple,
lime juice, maple syrup and coconut, especially when you then sprinkle granola on top.
This looks amazing presented in individual glass jars with the granola topping; the
layers really stand out and your friends and family will absolutely love them!*

Serves 6

NUT-FREE

1 mango
½ pineapple
3 tablespoons maple syrup
4 tablespoons coconut chips
finely grated zest and juice of
   2 unwaxed limes
400g coconut yogurt
3 passion fruits
220g granola, plus more to serve
   (page 29 for home-made)

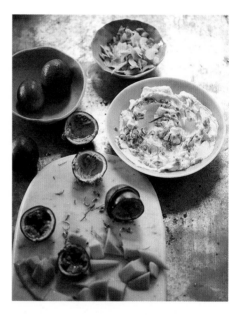

Start by peeling the mango and pineapple
and roughly chopping them into little pieces.

In a large mixing bowl, mix the mango,
pineapple, maple syrup, coconut chips and
lime zest and juice. Set aside to give time for
the flavours to mingle.

In a high-speed blender, whizz together the
coconut yogurt and the flesh of the passion
fruits until smooth, then put the mixture in the
fridge to chill.

Line up 6 jars, glasses or bowls and divide
the yogurt between them, then spoon a layer
of the fruit salad mix into each. Chill until
you want to serve, then take them out of the
fridge and sprinkle with granola.

CLEVER COOK
Don't add the granola too far in advance, or it
will become soggy.

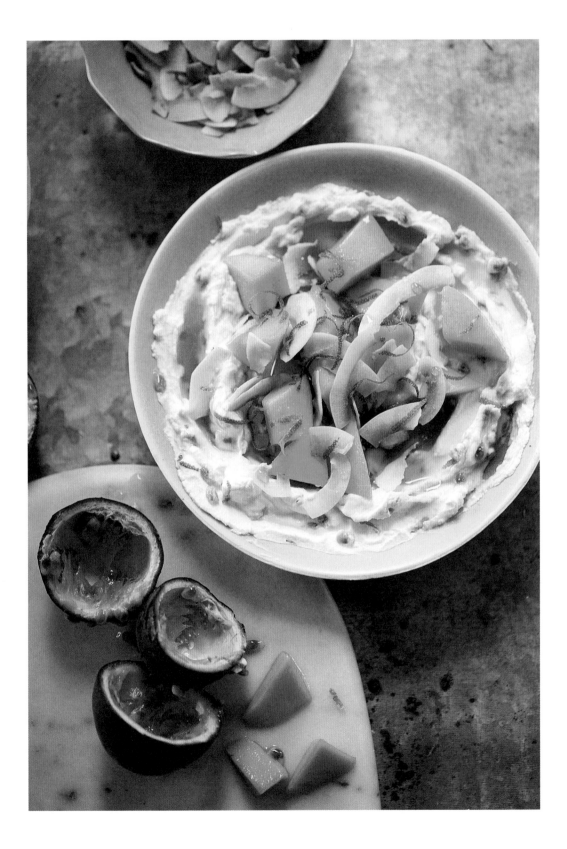

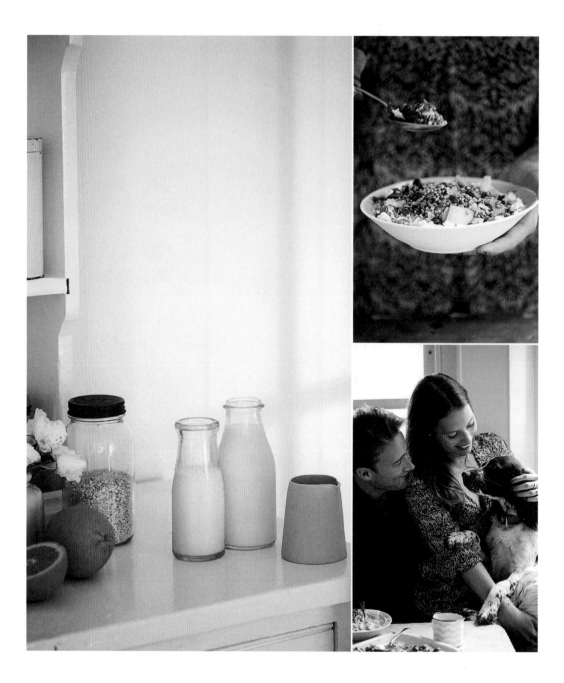

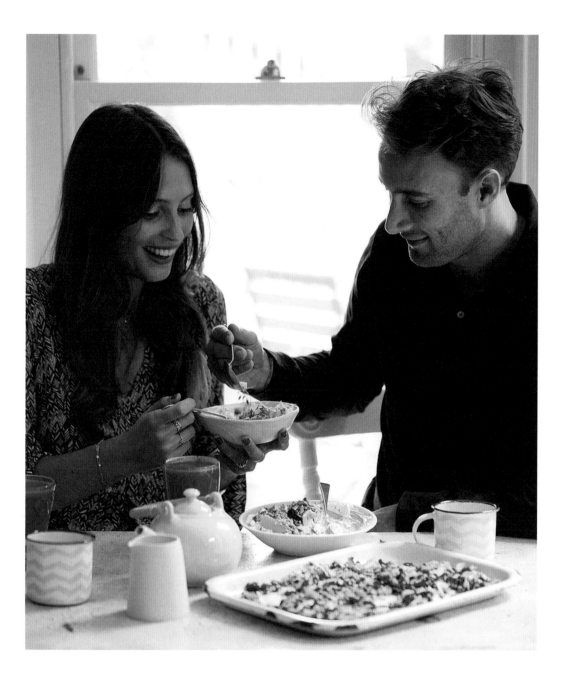

BLUEBERRY PANCAKE STACK

This was one of the first recipes I created for this book, and is still one of my favourites.
I started cooking these to fuel my running when I was training for a half marathon, and
they've become a weekend staple ever since. A thick stack of them is my dream breakfast,
especially when they're piled high with Caramelised Banana Bites, some extra maple
syrup and a big dollop of home-made Crunchy Cacao & Almond Butter
(pages 37 and 40). There's really nothing about these that tastes healthy,
they feel totally delicious and indulgent.

Makes about 12

NUT-FREE

2 tablespoons chia seeds

200g oats

2 over-ripe bananas, peeled

3 tablespoons maple syrup

2 tablespoons coconut oil,
    plus more to cook

pinch of salt

150g blueberries

Start by putting the chia seeds into a mug with 175ml of water. Let this sit for 20 minutes until the seeds expand and form a gel.

Place all the other ingredients, except the blueberries and the chia mixture, into a food processor with 100ml of water and blend until you have a smooth batter.

Transfer the mix to a bowl and stir in the blueberries, then the chia gel.

Oil a non-stick frying pan with a little coconut oil. Place over a high heat until it's really hot.

Now simply add 2 heaped tablespoons of batter to the pan for each pancake, use a spoon to shape into an even circle and let it cook for about 2 minutes per side, flipping it over once. Repeat for each pancake, until all the batter has been used, keeping them warm in a low oven until you're ready to eat.

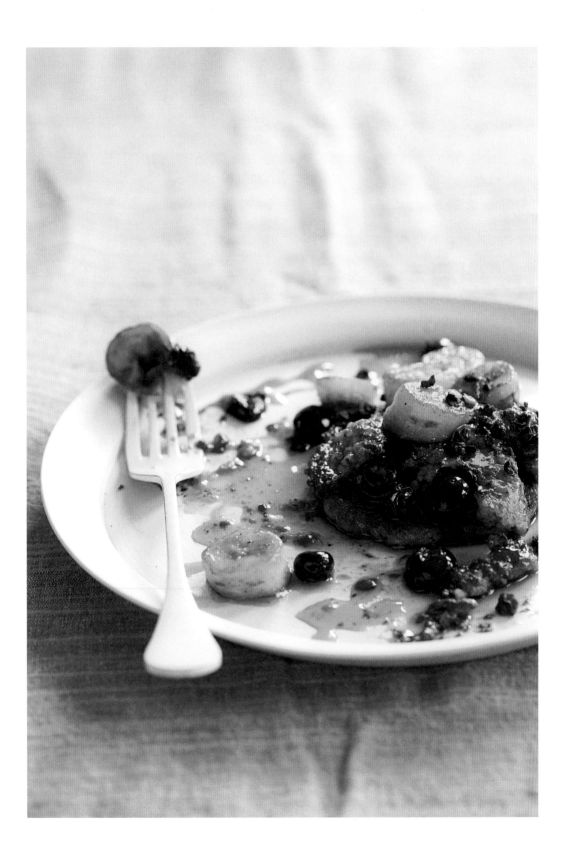

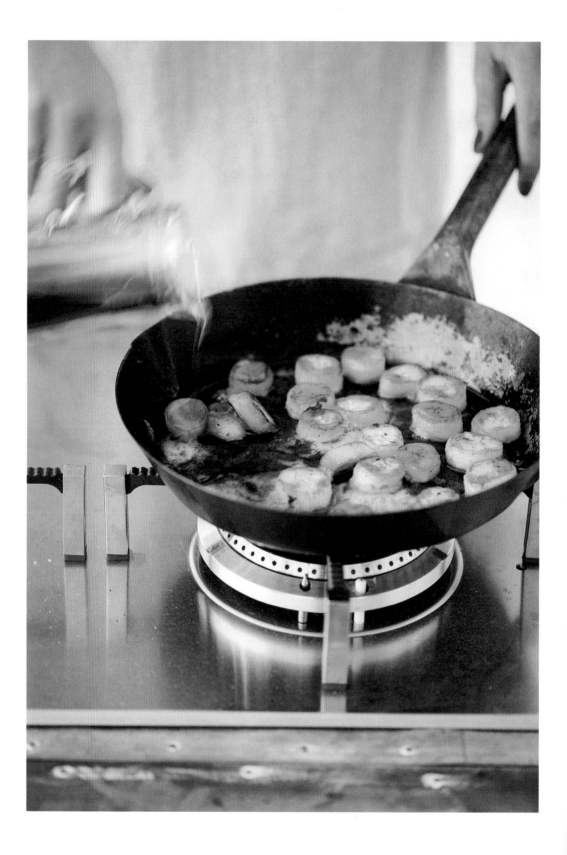

CARAMELISED BANANA BITES

I made these to enjoy with my Blueberry Pancake Stack (page 34), but loved them so much that I now try to sneak them into my breakfasts all the time. I love how they sizzle in the pan as you fry them, and you can smell the sweet coconut, cinnamon and maple flavours that they're absorbing — it's amazing — plus they're so quick to make. You have to try them with the pancakes, but also experiment by adding these to a simple porridge bowl: they'll instantly transform it into something really special.

Serves 4

NUT-FREE

4 bananas
1 tablespoon coconut oil
3 tablespoons maple syrup
1 teaspoon ground cinnamon

Slice the bananas a generous 2cm thick.

Heat a frying pan with the coconut oil, maple syrup and cinnamon over a medium-high heat until it is all really hot and bubbling. Add the banana slices; they should sizzle the moment they hit the pan.

Reduce the heat and cook for 2–3 minutes, stirring occasionally to make sure the slices are all fully coated and cooking evenly. When they're done they should be soft, gooey and coated in caramelised deliciousness!

PAN TO PLATE
10 minutes

CLEVER COOKING
If you're making these to serve with the pancakes (page 34), then just use the same pan to cook the bananas once you've finished making the pancakes. Cuts down on the washing-up!

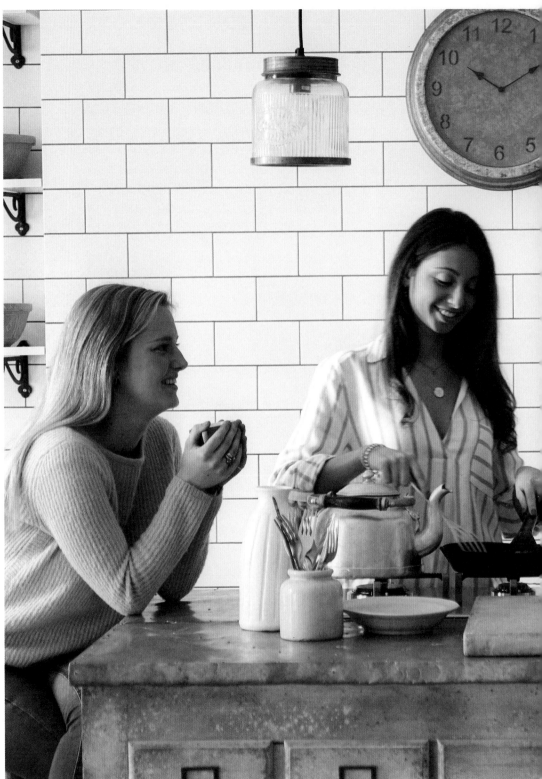

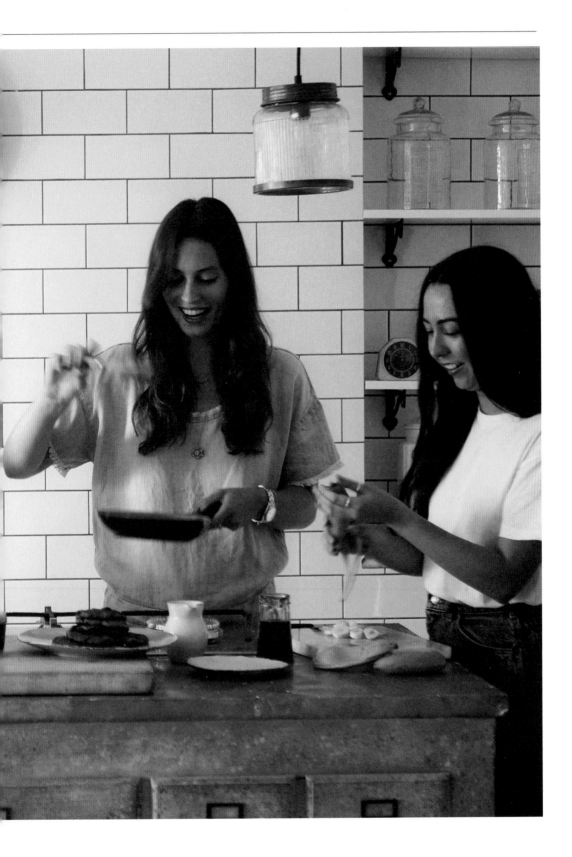

CRUNCHY CACAO & ALMOND BUTTER

Nut butter is a real staple in my life. I always have about ten open jars in my cupboard and at least one spoonful seems to somehow work its way into almost every meal I eat! This is my favourite for breakfast, though, it's got a lovely subtle sweetness from the vanilla, while the cacao nibs give it a great little crunch. Dollop this on pancake stacks, stir it into porridge bowls, spread it on toast, blend it into smoothies or just spoon it straight from the jar!

Makes 1 jar

300g almonds
generous pinch of salt
4 teaspoons cacao nibs
3 teaspoons raw cacao powder
2 teaspoons date syrup
2 teaspoons vanilla powder

Preheat the oven to 200°C (fan 180°C). Spread the almonds over a baking tray in a single layer and bake for 10 minutes. Keep an eye on them and don't let them burn, as this will ruin the flavours.

Let the almonds cool, then blend with the salt in a powerful food processor for about 10 minutes to form a smooth, creamy paste.

Scrape the almond butter from the blender into a large mixing bowl and stir in all the other ingredients. (Stirring these in, rather than blending, creates a smoother texture.)

Store in an airtight container for up to 5 days.

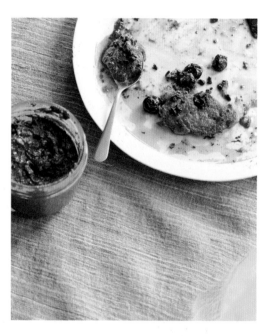

CLEVER COOKING
Make sure the almonds are fresh. All nuts can turn rancid quite quickly in the cupboard, which really affects the taste.

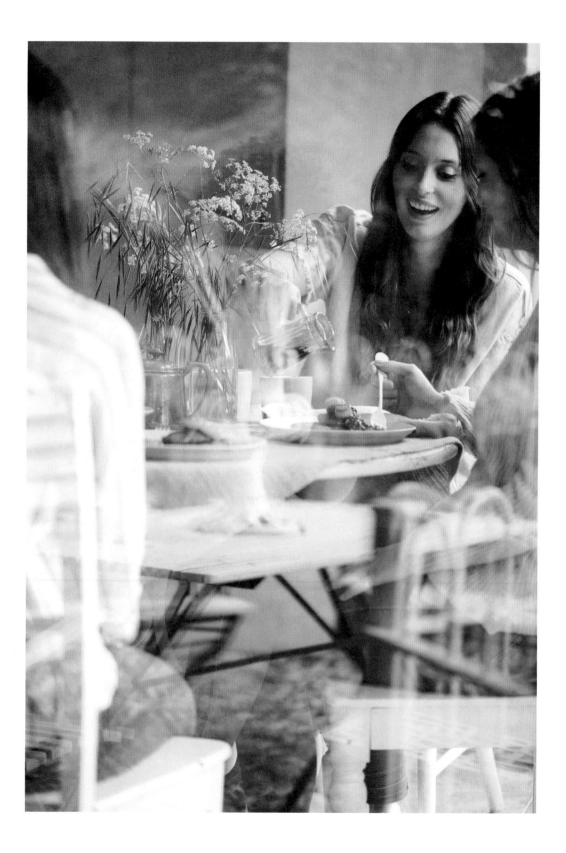

SCRAMBLED TURMERIC & RED PEPPER TOFU

Scrambled tofu might sound really weird, but trust me, it's so worth trying! It makes a lovely breakfast, especially with hot Thyme Fried Mushrooms, Garlicky Baked Tomatoes (pages 45 and 46) and some toasted rye bread spread with a thick layer of smashed avocado.

Serves 4

NUT-FREE

olive oil

1 red pepper, deseeded and
   finely chopped

6 spring onions

20g chives

1 tablespoon nutritional yeast

salt and pepper

1 tablespoon tamari

1 teaspoon ground turmeric

juice of ½ lemon

400g firm tofu (ideally organic)

PAN TO PLATE

15 minutes

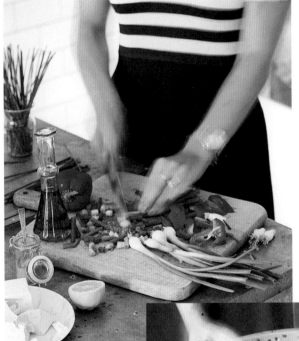

Heat a glug of olive oil in a frying pan and cook the pepper for 4–5 minutes.

Meanwhile, finely slice the spring onions and chives. Stir the spring onions into the peppers and cook for another minute before adding the chives, nutritional yeast, salt and pepper, tamari, turmeric and lemon juice. Finally, crumble in the tofu.

Cook for another 5 minutes until the tofu is hot, stirring every now and again.

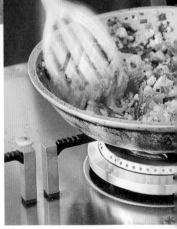

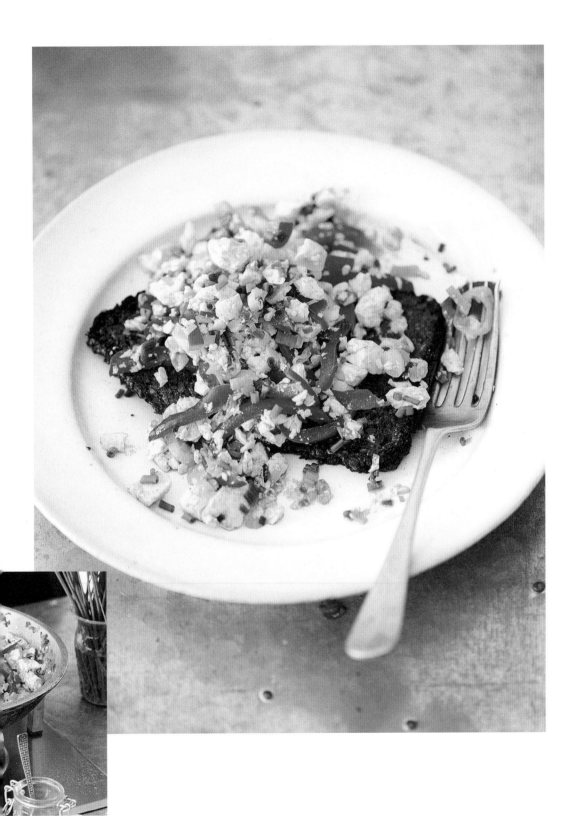

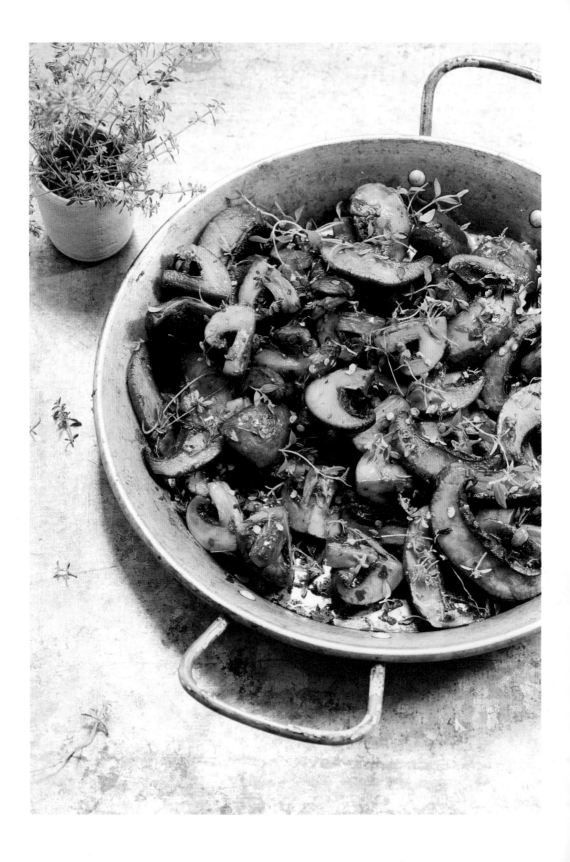

THYME FRIED MUSHROOMS

These are a weekend staple in our house. They're simple to make but bursting with flavour, and make any meal extra-satisfying and hearty. I love piling these on to a piece of rye toast with Garlicky Baked Tomatoes (page 46), or using them as a side for a quinoa bowl later in the day.

Serves 4

NUT-FREE

2 garlic cloves, crushed

salt and pepper

olive oil

a few sprigs of fresh thyme

1 teaspoon brown rice miso paste

½ teaspoon chilli flakes

6 Portobello mushrooms, thickly sliced

350g chestnut mushrooms, halved or quartered, depending on size

Place the garlic, salt and pepper in a large frying pan with a glug of olive oil. Let this heat for a few minutes, until it starts bubbling.

Now throw in the thyme and add the miso paste, chilli and all the mushrooms. Keep stirring the mushrooms until they release their juices, then let the pan simmer over a low heat until most of the juices evaporate.

After about 10 minutes they should be cooked perfectly. Remove from the heat and grind over a good amount of black pepper. Eat straight away.

PAN TO PLATE
15 minutes

GARLICKY BAKED TOMATOES

This is a wonderfully simple dish. I find tomatoes often taste best when left mostly untouched, as their natural flavour and juicy texture are really special, especially when baked. Adding the garlic, basil and apple cider vinegar does heighten their natural taste though, which is lovely. An easy addition to any savoury breakfast.

Serves 4

NUT-FREE

4 large vine tomatoes

2 tablespoons olive oil

lots of salt and pepper

6 garlic cloves, peeled

350g cherry tomatoes, preferably
on the vine

2 tablespoons apple cider vinegar

small handful of basil leaves

Preheat the oven to 200°C (fan 180°C).

While the oven heats up, cut the vine tomatoes in half. Place them flat sides down in a baking tray and drizzle with the olive oil. Grind in lots of salt and pepper and throw in the whole garlic cloves.

Bake in the oven for 30 minutes.

Take the tomatoes out of the oven and add the cherry tomatoes and vinegar. Reduce the oven temperature to 180°C (fan 160°C) and bake all the tomatoes together for another 40–45 minutes.

Roughly chop or tear the basil and sprinkle over the tomatoes and garlic before serving.

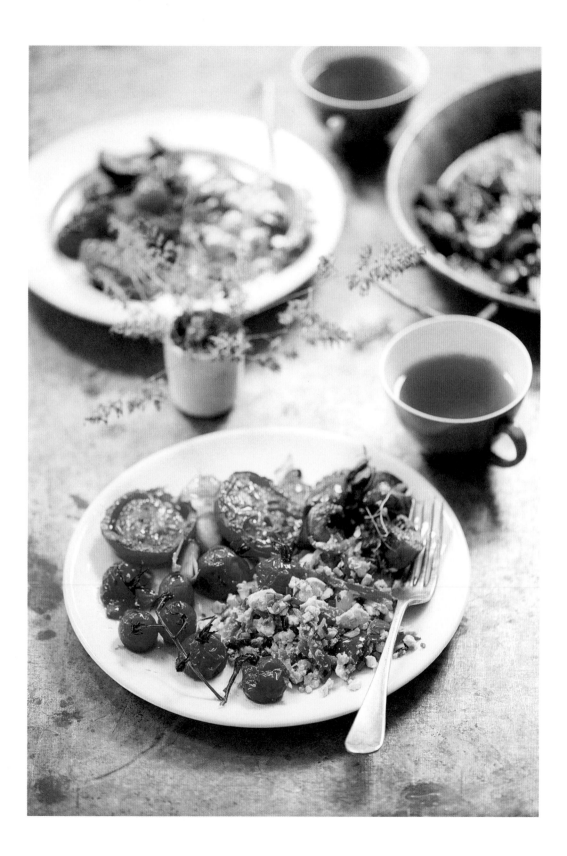

SWEET POTATO ROSTI

*A great base for a big breakfast. I love spreading a thick layer of my Herby Guacamole
on top of these, then piling them high with hot Maple & Rosemary Butter Beans
(pages 52 and 51). It makes for a really beautiful, hearty and delicious brunch.*

Serves 2

NUT-FREE

4 tablespoons olive oil

1 sweet potato, peeled and grated

1 red chilli, deseeded and finely chopped
(if you like it less spicy, only use ½ chilli)

1 tablespoon sesame seeds

4 tablespoons buckwheat flour

salt and pepper

In a large, non-stick lidded frying pan, heat
2 tablespoons of the oil over a high heat.

Meanwhile, place the remaining ingredients
in a bowl and mix them thoroughly.

Spoon the sweet potato mixture into the hot
oil, in 4 even mounds, making sure they're
not touching each other. Cook over a high
heat for about 2 minutes, gently pressing the
mixture down every now and again so that
they compress into nicely shaped patties.

Cover the pan and reduce the heat to as low
as it will go. Let the steam cook the patties
through for about 7 minutes. When you take
the lid off, the underside of the rostis should
be lovely and crispy and the patties will have
reduced in size.

Gently turn the rostis over with a spatula,
then whack the heat up to high again and
cook for 3 minutes until the second side is
browned nicely. Take off the heat and serve.

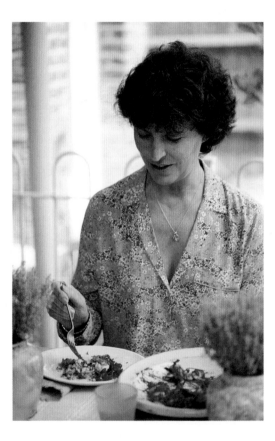

PAN TO PLATE

20 minutes

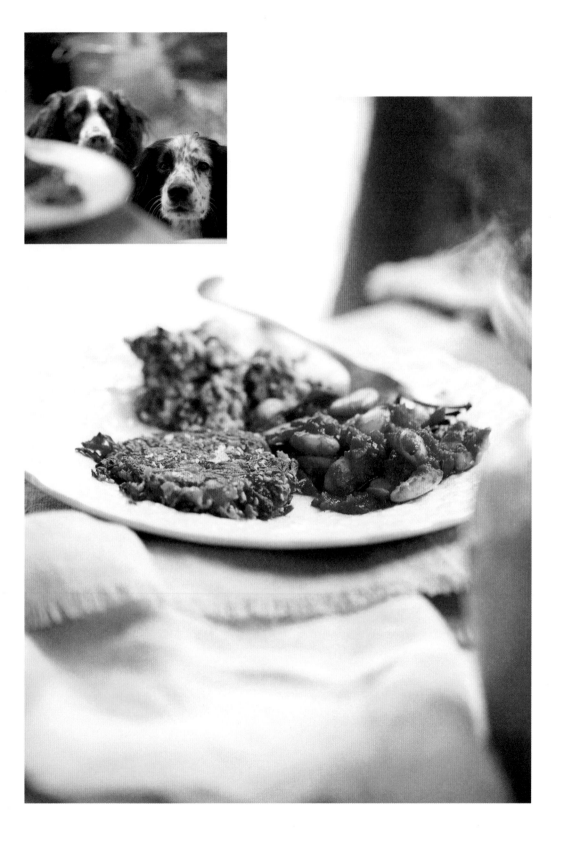

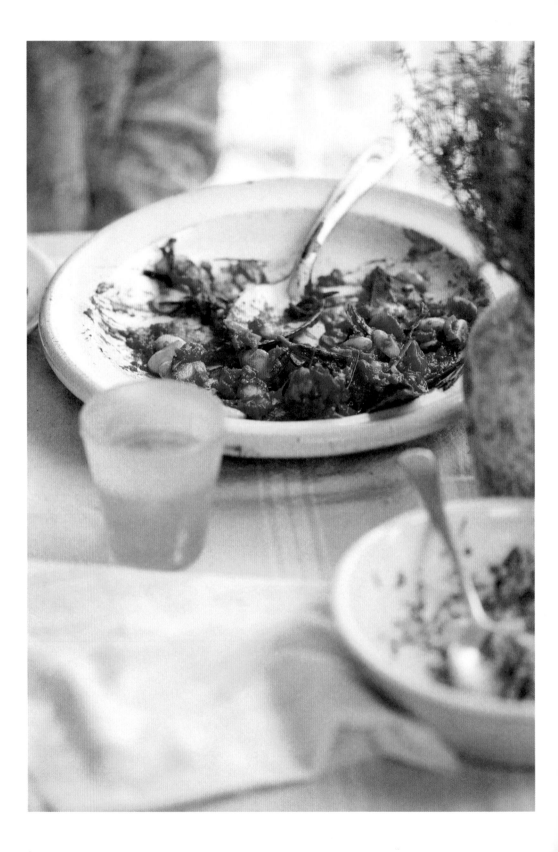

MAPLE & ROSEMARY BUTTER BEANS

*In our house, we seem to find ways to include these in breakfast, lunch and dinner!
They're so versatile and go with just about everything, although they are especially good
in this brunch combination. I just love how simple and yet how flavoursome they are.*

Serves 2

NUT-FREE

olive oil

3 garlic cloves, finely chopped

3 sprigs of fresh rosemary

1 bay leaf

½ teaspoon cayenne pepper

1 teaspoon smoked paprika

130g canned chopped tomatoes (about ⅓ can)

1 tablespoon maple syrup

1 tablespoon tomato purée

400g can of butter beans, drained and rinsed

salt and pepper

Preheat the oven to 180°C (fan 160°C).

Use an ovenproof casserole dish with a lid for this dish. Heat up a glug of olive oil and fry the garlic over a medium heat until it turns translucent but doesn't colour. Once this happens, add the herbs and spices, tomatoes, maple syrup and tomato purée, the beans, salt and pepper. Bring to the boil.

Once it starts to boil, clamp the lid on, turn the gas off and put the pan in the oven to bake for 30 minutes.

Remove the bay leaf and rosemary stalks before serving (the rosemary leaves will have dropped off into the beans) and enjoy.

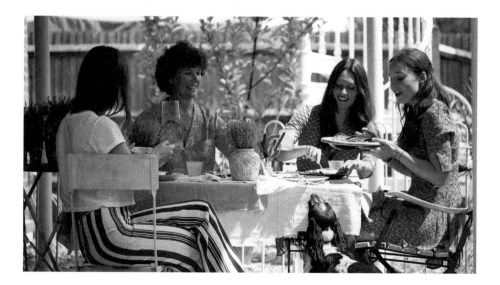

HERBY GUACAMOLE

*Probably my favourite part of this brunch, with the rosti and butter beans (pages 48
and 51). I find that the creamy texture really brings the other two dishes together.
The avocado is mixed with a beautiful blend of roughly chopped aromatic basil,
coriander, mint and parsley, to create something that's just bursting with flavour;
I'm sure all you avocado fans will absolutely love it! It's a great addition to any meal and
an easy snack to keep in the fridge. I adore piling it on to a slice of rye toast for breakfast,
using it as a dip for a quick snack, or adding it to a big quinoa bowl.*

Serves 2

NUT-FREE

2 avocados

1 tablespoon olive oil

juice of 1 lime

6g fresh basil leaves, roughly chopped

6g fresh coriander leaves,
    roughly chopped

3g fresh mint leaves, roughly chopped

3g fresh parsley leaves,
    roughly chopped

lots of salt and pepper

Pit and peel the avocados, then mash
them in a bowl with a fork.

Stir in all the rest of the ingredients. This is
best served fresh. It won't keep for more
than a day or so and the herbs will start to
turn brown.

SUPER-SPEEDY

10 minutes

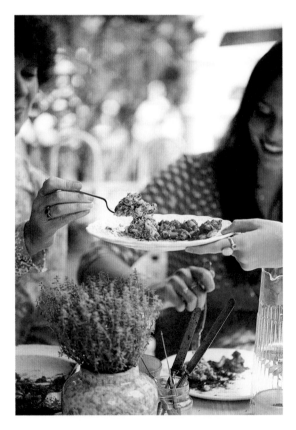

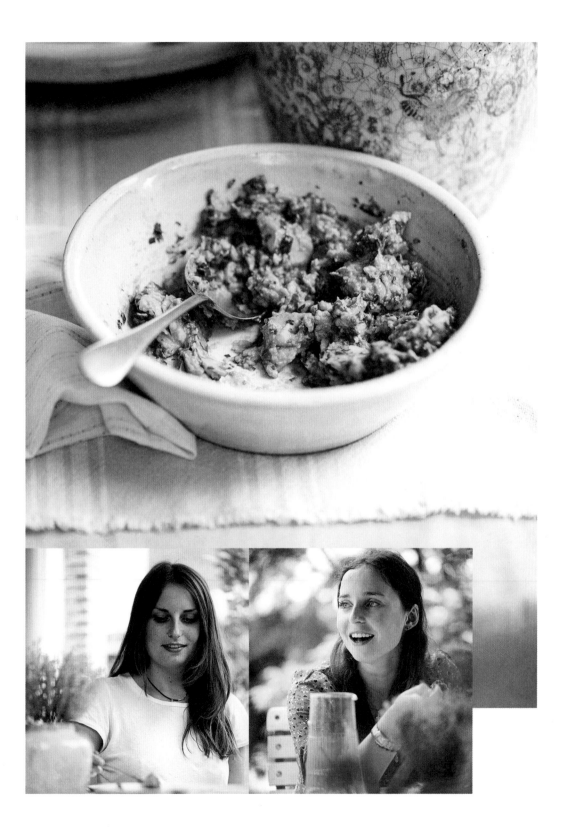

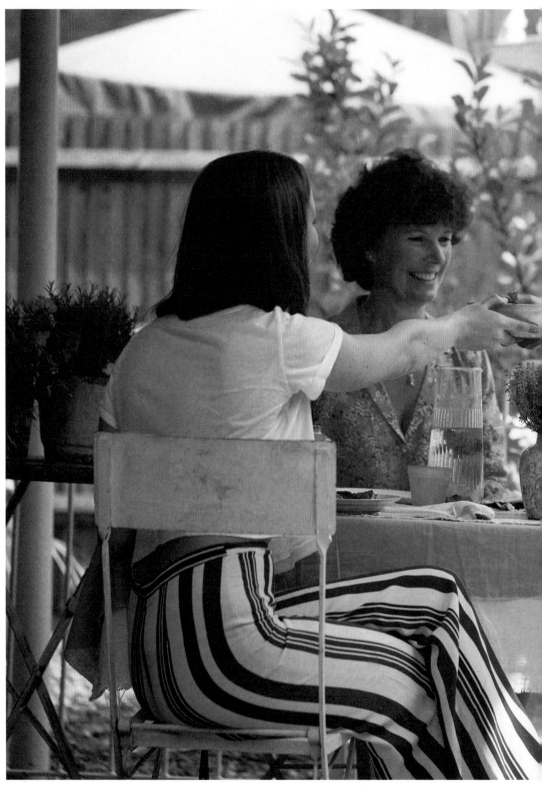

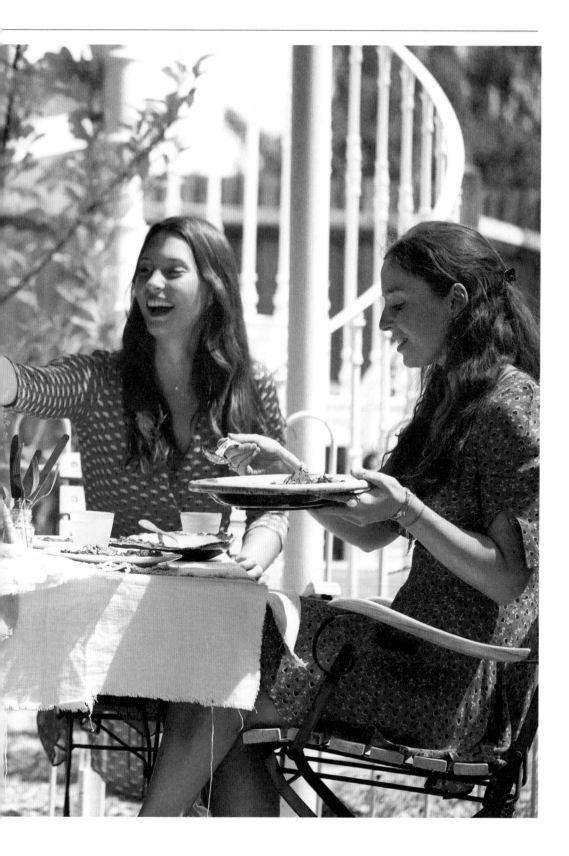

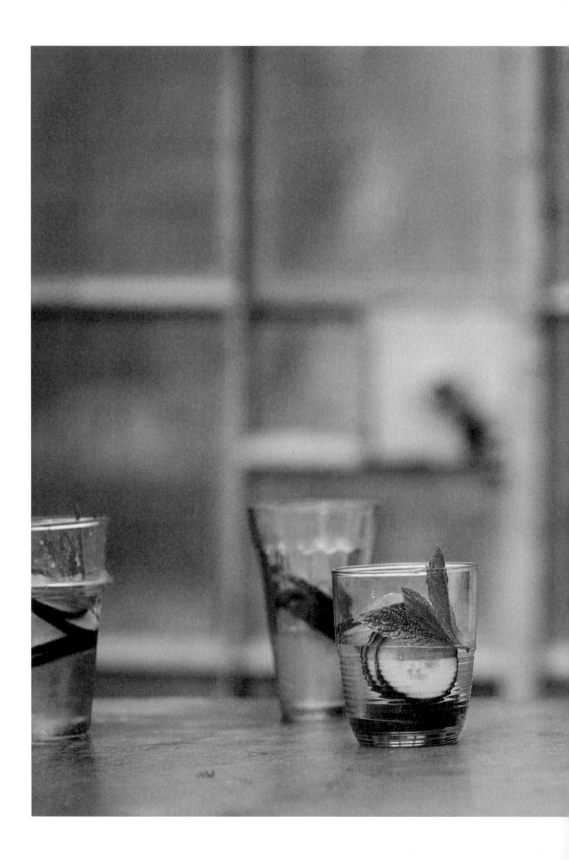

LIGHT & EASY

QUICK MEALS TO NOURISH YOUR BODY & FEED YOUR FRIENDS

LIGHT & EASY

This is probably the chapter of the book that I use the most at home. It's packed with simple recipes that you can make and share every day, to keep you and the people around you feeling happy and healthy. It's hard to pick favourites from these recipes, as I genuinely love and use them all, but I would recommend a plate of hot Spiced Potato Cakes with Garlicky Tomato Sauce on a bed of French Beans with Tomato if you want something nourishing and warming, or the Mango & Mushroom Ceviche if you want something lighter and more refreshing. Or, if you're looking for an upgrade to your lunch box, or to put together a simple picnic to share with a friend, try the Kale, Sun-dried Tomato, Olive & Sweet Potato Salad with Baked Sweet Potato & Sesame Falafels and maybe a side of hummus.

MENUS

AFTER-WORK CATCH-UP
Spiced Potato Cakes with Garlicky Tomato Sauce
French Beans with Tomato

FRESH BITES
Mango & Mushroom Ceviche
Cauli Rice, Sesame & Beet Nigiri Sushi

AL DESKO
Baked Sweet Potato & Sesame Falafels
Kale, Sun-dried Tomato, Olive & Sweet Potato Salad

PERFECT PICNIC
Charred Coconut Corn
Pepper, Mango, Cucumber & Peanut Salad

STORECUPBOARD SAVIOUR
Lemony Potato & Butter Bean Salad
Baked Sesame & Tomato Avocados

COMFORT & SPICE
Sweet Potato Noodles with a Creamy Peanut Satay Sauce
Sautéed Tamari Greens

ASIAN-STYLE SUPPER
Chilli & Ginger Pho
Sesame & Maple Summer Rolls with Sweet Almond Dipping Sauce

SUMMER SALADS
Pistachio & Apricot Quinoa
Sesame Slaw

MIDWEEK PICK-ME-UP
Sautéed Tempeh with Roasted Garlic & Almond Pesto
Sesame, Coriander & Roasted Fennel Rice Bowl

SPICED POTATO CAKES WITH GARLICKY TOMATO SAUCE

These make an excellent weekday dinner. They're easy to make and so comforting after a long day at work, especially when covered in piping hot garlicky tomato sauce and served on a bed of French beans that echo their flavours (page 65). The potato cakes have so much flavour themselves, with their warming mix of spices and lemon, which adds a lovely freshness. Freeze any leftover cakes.

Makes 8 / Serves 4

NUT-FREE

FOR THE POTATO CAKES

750g potatoes (I use Maris Piper)

salt and pepper

3 tablespoons olive oil, plus more to cook

1 red chilli, deseeded and finely chopped, plus more to serve

2 garlic cloves, crushed

1 teaspoon ground cumin

1 teaspoon paprika

1 teaspoon ground turmeric

1 teaspoon chilli powder

20g fresh coriander, roughly chopped, plus more to serve

juice of 1 lemon

FOR THE SAUCE

750g cherry tomatoes, quartered

3 tablespoons olive oil

4 garlic cloves, crushed

salt and pepper

1 teaspoon chilli flakes (optional)

Peel the potatoes, quarter them, then place them in a saucepan of water with a pinch of salt. Bring to the boil and simmer for 20–25 minutes until cooked. Drain and leave to cool.

Meanwhile, heat the 3 tablespoons of oil in a frying pan, add the chilli and garlic and cook for a minute or so. Add the dry spices, sizzle for 30 seconds, then take off the heat. Preheat the oven to 200°C (fan 180°C).

Once the potatoes have cooled, add all the remaining ingredients. Mix until smooth, then shape into 8 patties. Place on a baking tray. Drizzle with olive oil. Bake for 25–30 minutes, turning halfway, until they are golden brown.

Meanwhile, make the sauce. Simply throw all the ingredients into a saucepan and simmer for about 20 minutes, until the tomatoes have cooked down and the sauce is rich and thick.

Serve the potato cakes with the sauce, sprinkling with fresh coriander and chilli, with the French Beans with Tomato (page 65).

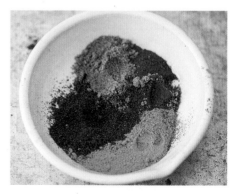

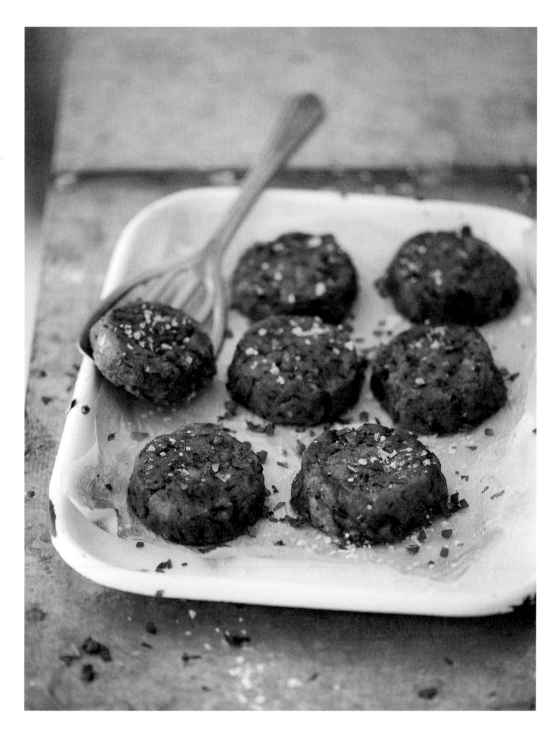

MIX IT UP

If you want to skip the tomato sauce, these potato cakes also
taste incredible with Coconut Tzatziki (page 209).

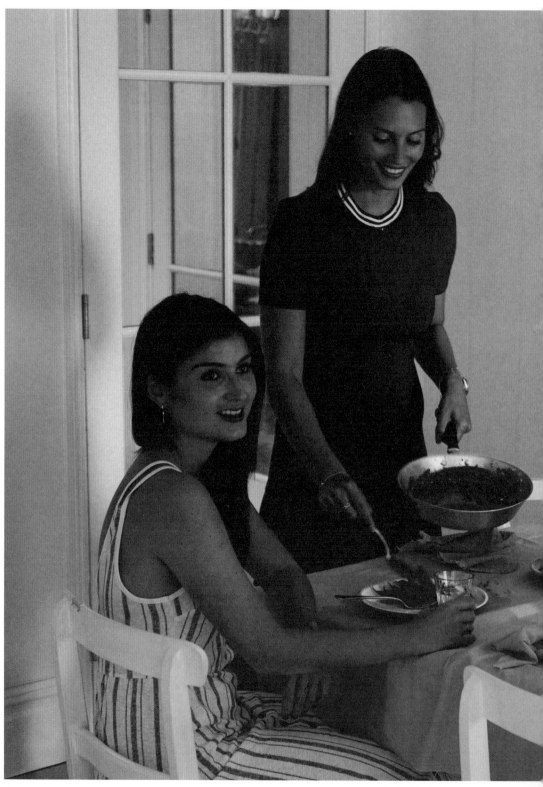

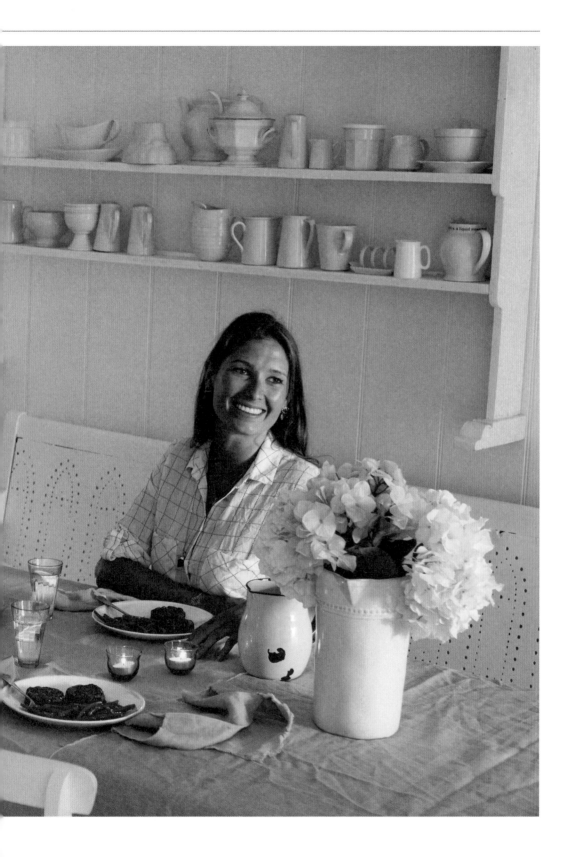

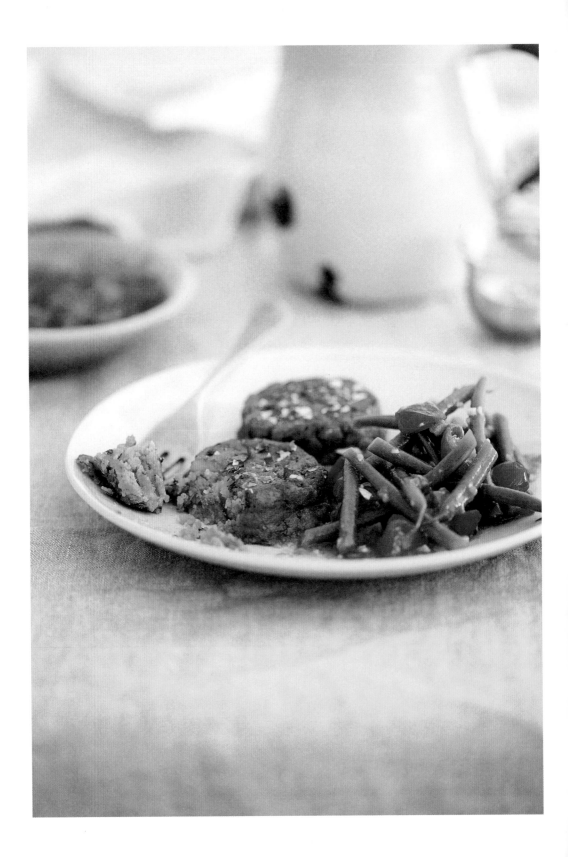

FRENCH BEANS WITH TOMATO

I love using these as a bed for my Spiced Potato Cakes with Garlicky Tomato Sauce (page 60), as the contrast of textures is so perfect. The lightly cooked beans have a lovely snap and crunch, while the potato cakes are soft and just melt in your mouth. The garlic and tomato in the beans really complements the sauce of the potatoes, too, creating a perfect meal. These French beans work as a great side with a host of other meals.

Serves 4 as a side dish

NUT-FREE

2 tablespoons olive oil

100g cherry tomatoes, quartered

3 garlic cloves, crushed

1 tablespoon apple cider vinegar

salt and pepper

200g French beans, tops trimmed, halved

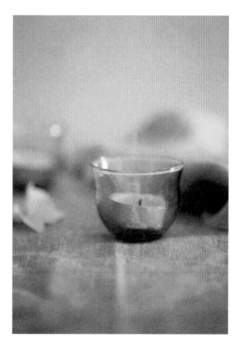

Heat the olive oil in a large sauté pan over a medium heat, then add the tomatoes and let them cook down until they start to disintegrate and caramelise. Meanwhile fill a kettle with water and bring it to the boil.

When the tomatoes are a rich red colour, after about 5 minutes, add in the garlic, vinegar and salt and pepper and cook for about 1 minute.

Meanwhile, pop the green beans into a sieve and pour the boiling water from the kettle over them so they start to soften, then put them into the pan with the tomato and garlic mixture.

Stir over the heat for a couple of minutes to heat through, season to taste, then serve.

PAN TO PLATE

15 minutes

MIX IT UP

Try stirring these through a bowl of penne pasta; it's absolutely delicious and a wonderfully quick meal.

MANGO & MUSHROOM CEVICHE

*I first had a mushroom ceviche at one of my favourite restaurants about a year ago
and have been in love with the dish ever since. It's wonderfully light, full of flavour and
incredibly refreshing. The mushrooms are marinated in an amazing mix of lime juice,
ginger, chilli and olive oil, then tossed with juicy bites of mango and crunchy red pepper,
which together taste incredible. The flavours only get stronger the longer you marinate
this, so make extra to enjoy as leftovers a few days later.*

Serves 4

NUT-FREE

400g button mushrooms, very thinly sliced
juice of 10 limes (about 150ml)
50ml olive oil
1 garlic clove, crushed
2.5cm root ginger, finely grated
1 jalapeño chilli, or other chilli,
    finely chopped
salt
⅓ red onion, finely chopped
1 red pepper, deseeded and finely chopped
¾ ripe mango, peeled, pitted and
    finely chopped
small handful of fresh coriander,
    roughly chopped

Place the mushrooms in a large bowl and
pour over the lime juice, olive oil, garlic,
ginger, chilli and salt to taste. Toss together
gently, cover and allow to marinate for about
1 hour at room temperature, for the flavours
to develop.

When you're ready to serve, stir in the onion,
pepper, mango and most of the coriander,
then arrange it on a serving platter. Sprinkle
on the remaining coriander when you serve,
to make it look even more beautiful.

Any leftovers will keep in an airtight container
in the fridge for up to 4 days.

SUPER-SPEEDY
10 minutes

MIX IT UP
Try topping this with the kernels cut from
Charred Coconut Corn (page 76), it tastes
amazing.

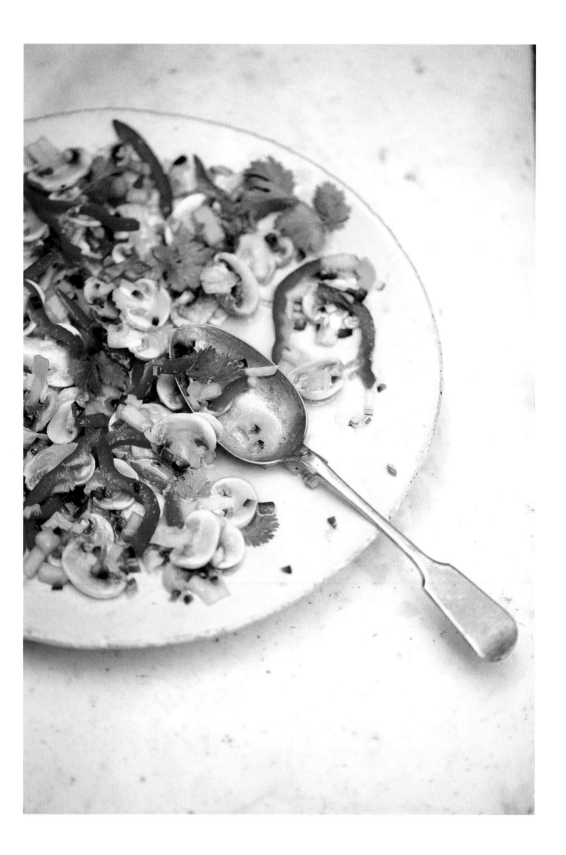

CAULI RICE, SESAME & BEET NIGIRI SUSHI

This veggie nigiri is a little unusual and it's a really lovely nibble. Using cauliflower rice makes a nice, light change from sushi rice, while the brightly coloured avocado and beet make it look fantastic. I love dipping these nigiri into the tamari, sesame and lime sauce, to deepen the flavours. You'll need a jelly bag to prepare the rice; find them online.

Makes 10 pieces

FOR THE 'RICE'

1 large cauliflower

1 tablespoon apple cider vinegar

1 tablespoon toasted sesame oil

1 tablespoon tamari

130ml coconut milk

salt

FOR THE AVOCADO CREAM

1 ripe avocado

1 tablespoon apple cider vinegar

1 tablespoon olive oil

FOR THE BEETROOT

1 cooked beetroot, peeled

FOR THE DIPPING SAUCE

1 tablespoon toasted sesame oil

2 tablespoons tamari

1 tablespoon sesame seeds,
    plus more to serve

juice of ½ lime

Cut the cauliflower florets from the stem and chop them into 2.5–5cm pieces. This will make 'ricing' them easier. Place in a food processor and pulse until it looks like rice; this takes about 30 seconds.

Place in a jelly bag and knead out excess water. This takes a few minutes as cauliflower contains a lot of water, it's a really important step though, so please don't skip it, or the rice won't hold together when you mould it.

Once most of the water has been removed, add the cauliflower to a saucepan with the remaining rice ingredients and heat for about 10 minutes, until the coconut milk has been absorbed and there is no liquid left in the pan. The rice should start to feel a bit sticky at this point. Put it into a sieve and press out any remaining liquid, then tip it out into a bowl and firmly press it down. Set aside.

Now make the avocado cream. Wash the food processor, then pit and peel the avocado and place it in the food processor with all the remaining avocado cream ingredients, adding 1 tablespoon of water and a little more salt. Blend until the mix is smooth and creamy. Set aside.

Very finely slice the beetroot.

To make the dipping sauce, simply mix all the ingredients together thoroughly.

Now assemble the nigiri. Mould together the cauliflower rice into little oblong nigiri shapes. Spoon a neat blob of the avocado cream on top and lay a thin slice of beetroot over the cream. Sprinkle with sesame seeds, then arrange on a serving platter with shallow bowls of the dipping sauce.

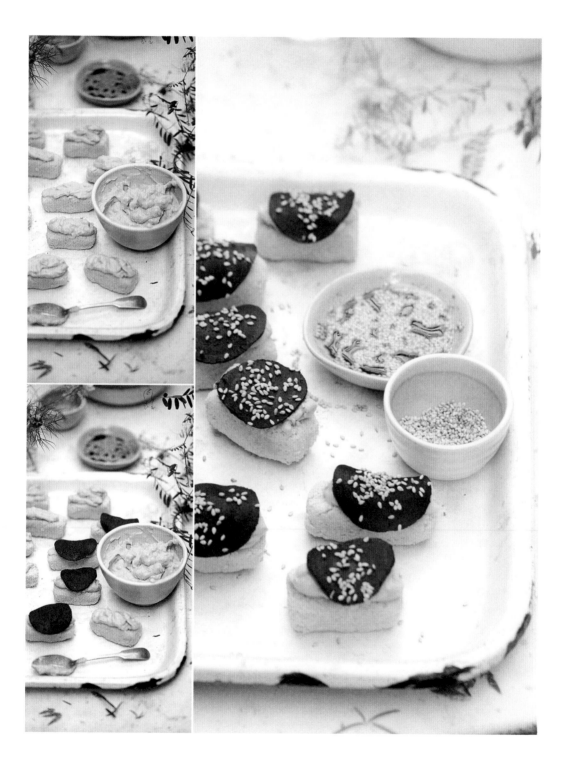

BAKED SWEET POTATO & SESAME FALAFELS

These are such a great addition to an on-the-go lunch box. They're quick and simple to make and freeze well, too, so you can build a stash in the freezer to keep you fuelled throughout the week. I love the sesame seeds on the outside, it gives such a lovely crunch and makes them look beautiful. They also travel really easily, making them a great al desko lunch, so I'm sure lots of your colleagues will be very jealous! They taste amazing with Kale, Sun-dried Tomato, Olive & Sweet Potato Salad (page 75), the contrasting textures are perfect together.

Makes 14

NUT-FREE

FOR THE SWEET POTATO PURÉE

2 sweet potatoes, peeled and
    roughly chopped

FOR THE FALAFELS

4 garlic cloves, roughly chopped

handful of fresh coriander, chopped

4 tablespoons olive oil

juice of 1 lemon

2 teaspoons ground cumin

2 teaspoons smoked paprika

1 teaspoon ground turmeric

2 teaspoons apple cider vinegar

½ teaspoon cayenne pepper

2 tablespoons tahini

salt and pepper

3 tablespoons gram (chickpea) flour

2 x 400g cans of chickpeas,
    drained and rinsed

100g sesame seeds

Steam the sweet potatoes for 30 minutes, or until completely soft. Blend for a few seconds to make a smooth purée.

Preheat the oven to 220°C (fan 200°C). Line 1 large baking sheet, or 2 medium-sized baking sheets, with baking parchment.

Put all the ingredients for the falafels, except the chickpeas and sesame seeds, into a food processor, add 14 tablespoons of the sweet potato purée and blend until almost smooth, then season really well, add the chickpeas and pulse a few times to form a chunky mix.

Tip the sesame seeds on to a plate.

With wet hands, roll 1 heaped dessertspoon of the mix into a ball, roll it in the sesame seeds and place it on a baking tray. Keep going until all the mixture is used up.

Place the tray or trays into the oven and bake for 35–40 minutes. Leave to cool for 5 minutes on a wire rack before eating.

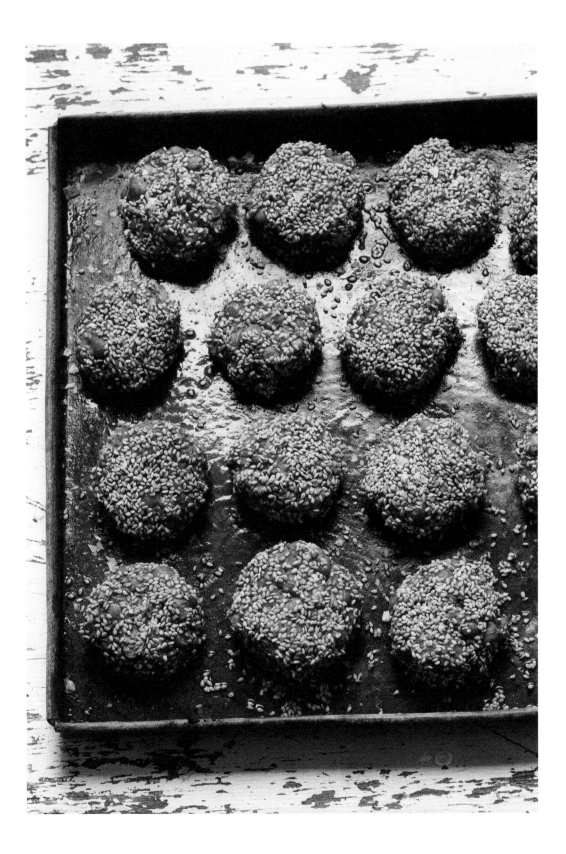

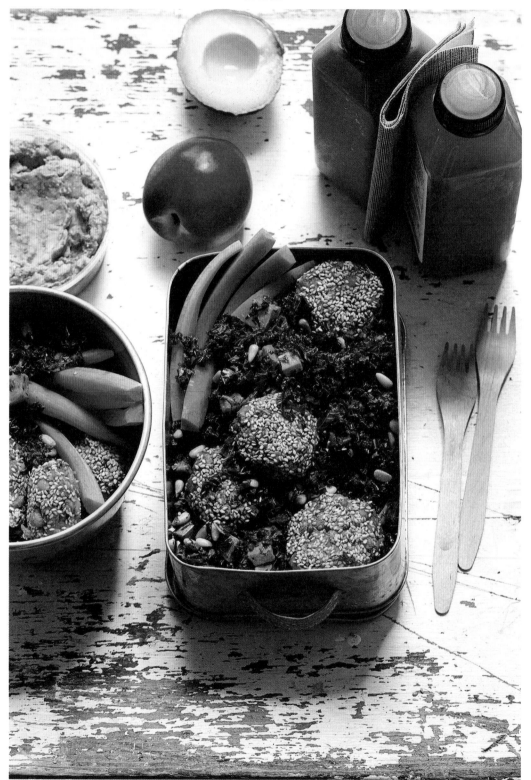

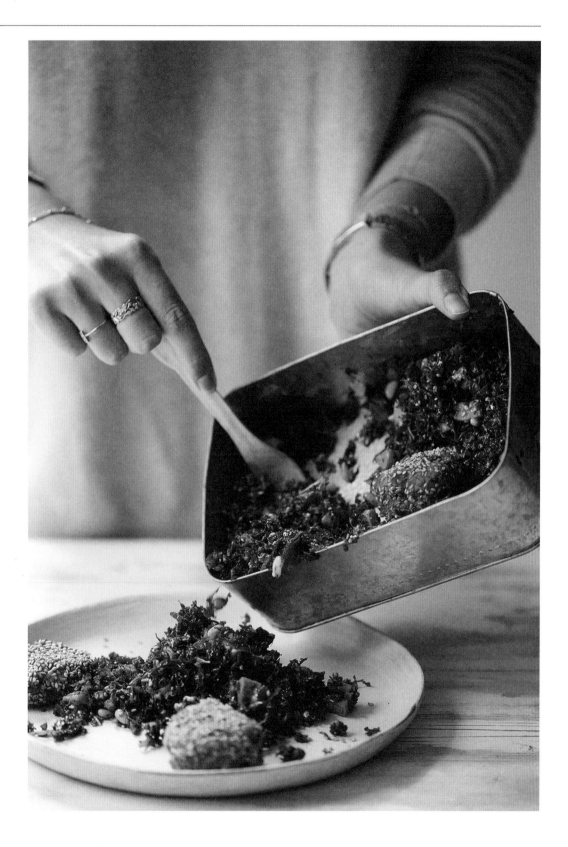

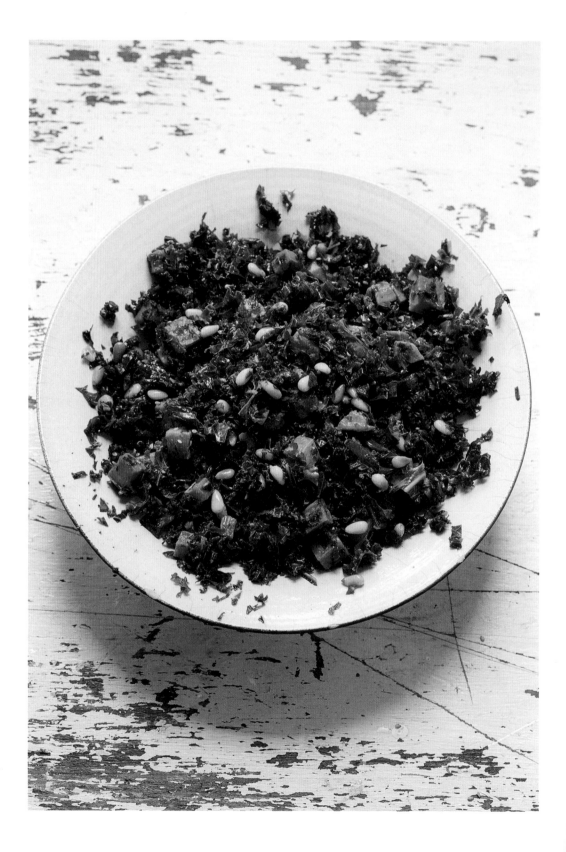

KALE, SUN-DRIED TOMATO, OLIVE & SWEET POTATO SALAD

A lovely chopped salad, filled with little bites of sweet potato, sun-dried tomatoes, black olives and toasted pine nuts, all tossed together with a simple olive oil, lemon and vinegar dressing. Its simplicity means it goes with just about everything, it's a perfect side salad for every meal! I particularly love it coupled with Baked Sweet Potato & Sesame Falafels though (page 70), they make a fantastic desk lunch, especially with a generous dollop of hummus or guacamole.

Serves 4

NUT-FREE

1 large sweet potato, peeled or
  well scrubbed
5 tablespoons olive oil
salt and pepper
200g kale, coarse ribs removed
2 tablespoons apple cider vinegar
juice of ½ lemon
100g sun-dried tomatoes in oil (drained
  weight), finely chopped
100g pitted black olives, finely chopped
100g pine nuts

Preheat the oven to 220°C (fan 200°C).

Cut the sweet potato into 1cm cubes, place in a roasting tray, drizzle with 2 tablespoons of the olive oil and add lots of salt and pepper. Roast for 45 minutes or until cooked through and slightly crispy.

Meanwhile, add the kale to a food processor and pulse a few times to break it down into little pieces. Tip it into a large salad bowl with the remaining olive oil, the vinegar, salt and pepper, the lemon juice, sun-dried tomatoes and olives. Toss the salad well so all the ingredients are evenly coated in the dressing.

When the sweet potato chunks are cooked, remove from the oven and stir them through the salad.

Finally, heat a frying pan over a medium heat and dry-fry the pine nuts for a few minutes, or until golden brown. (Watch carefully when cooking these, as they burn easily.) Remove from the heat and sprinkle on to the salad.

This tastes delicious warm or cold.

CHARRED COCONUT CORN

My family have an obsession with coconut corn, we've been eating it non-stop every summer for the last few years. There's something so delicious about the lightly charred corn kernels being coated in sweet coconut oil and salt, it's so addictive! They're amazing made in a pan, but if you can put them on the barbecue then they're even better.

Serves 4

NUT-FREE
coconut oil
4 heads of corn on the cob
salt

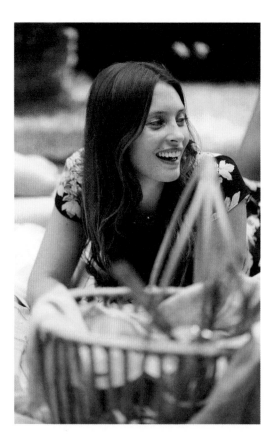

Put a griddle pan on the heat with a couple of tablespoons of coconut oil and get it nice and hot. Open the kitchen windows and doors and put on the extractor fan or – even better – cook it outdoors.

Add the corn cobs. You want to blacken some of the kernels, so leave the cob well alone for about a minute before you roll it on to another side, making sure you use some tongs, not fingers! Keep doing this until the corn cob is a nice mixture of black and yellow all round, then remove it and let it cool a little.

Sprinkle with salt and eat.

MIX IT UP
Try cutting the corn kernels off the cob and sprinkling them over Mango & Mushroom Ceviche (page 66); the two recipes taste amazing together!

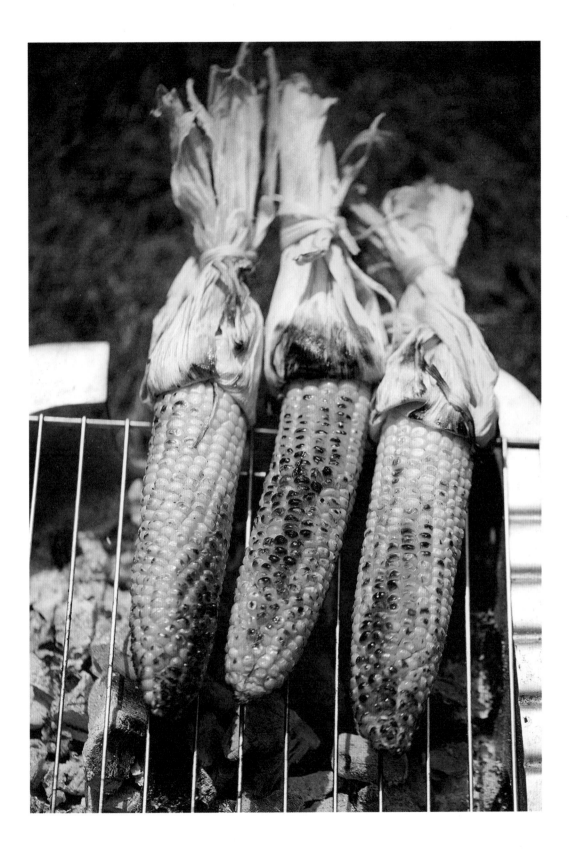

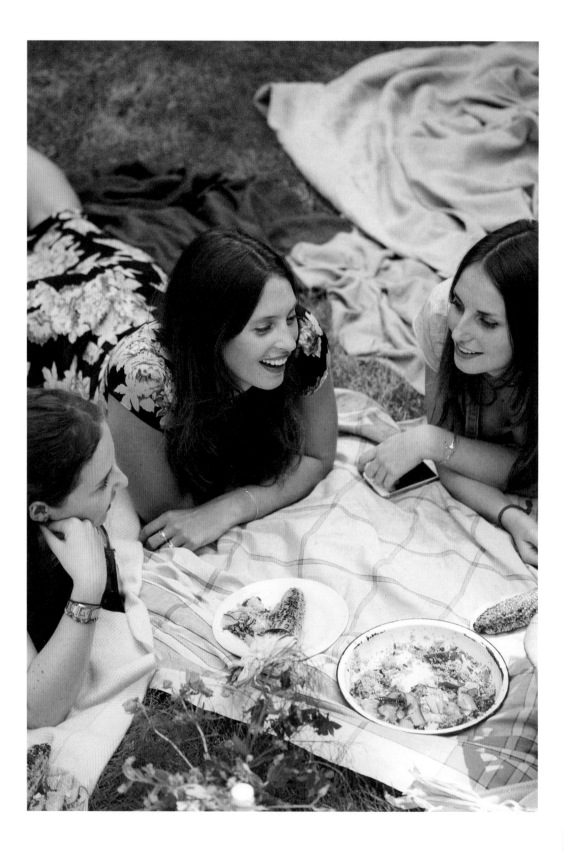

PEPPER, MANGO, CUCUMBER & PEANUT SALAD

A lovely summer lunch. The mango gives each bite a lovely sweetness, while the peanuts and sesame add great texture and flavour. It tastes amazing with kernels of Charred Coconut Corn (page 76) sprinkled across it, too!

Serves 4

FOR THE SALAD

100g raw, unsalted peanuts

2 tablespoons sesame seeds

1 red pepper, deseeded and finely sliced

4 garlic cloves, bashed, skins left on

olive oil

120g quinoa

1 small cucumber, shaved into ribbons
   with a peeler

½ red chilli, deseeded and finely chopped

1 mango, peeled, pitted and finely chopped

FOR THE DRESSING

2 tablespoons apple cider vinegar

2 tablespoons tamari

2 tablepoons toasted sesame oil

1 tablespoon peanut butter

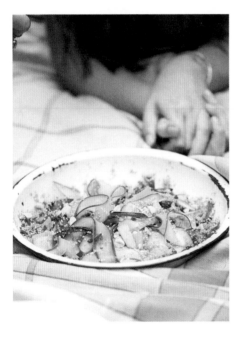

Preheat the oven to 200°C (fan 180°C). Place the peanuts on a baking tray and roast for 4 minutes. Take the tray out, give the peanuts a shake, then add the sesame seeds and pop them back in the oven for another 4 minutes, or until nicely browned. Set aside to cool.

Tumble the sliced red pepper on to another baking tray with the garlic cloves, drizzle with olive oil and put into the oven to cook for 20 minutes, giving them a shake halfway through; they should be soft by the time they come out of the oven.

Meanwhile, cook the quinoa. Put it into a saucepan with 250ml of water, bring to the boil and simmer for 12–15 minutes until all the water is absorbed, then set aside to cool. Mix the quinoa and roasted red pepper in a large salad bowl. Pick out the roasted garlic, peel and finely slice it, then stir it in, too. Mix all the ingredients for the dressing.

When you're ready to eat, simply add the peanuts and sesame seeds, cucumber, red chilli and mango, give it a gentle toss with the dressing, then devour.

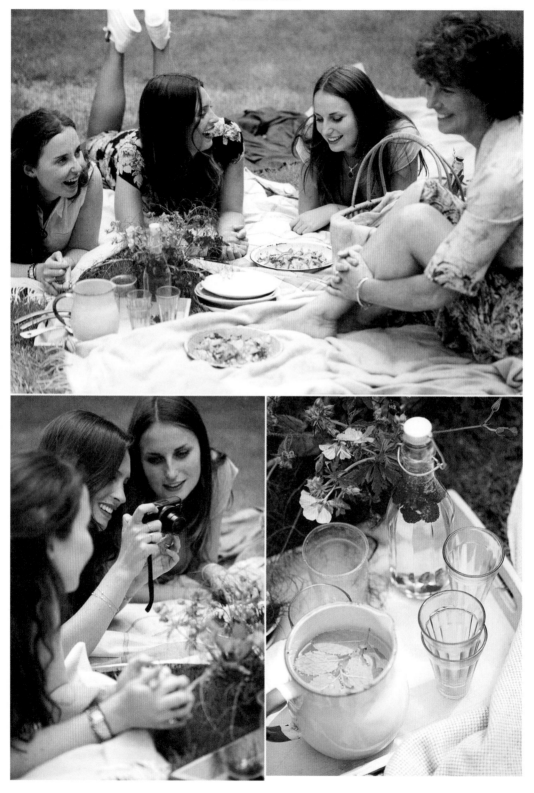

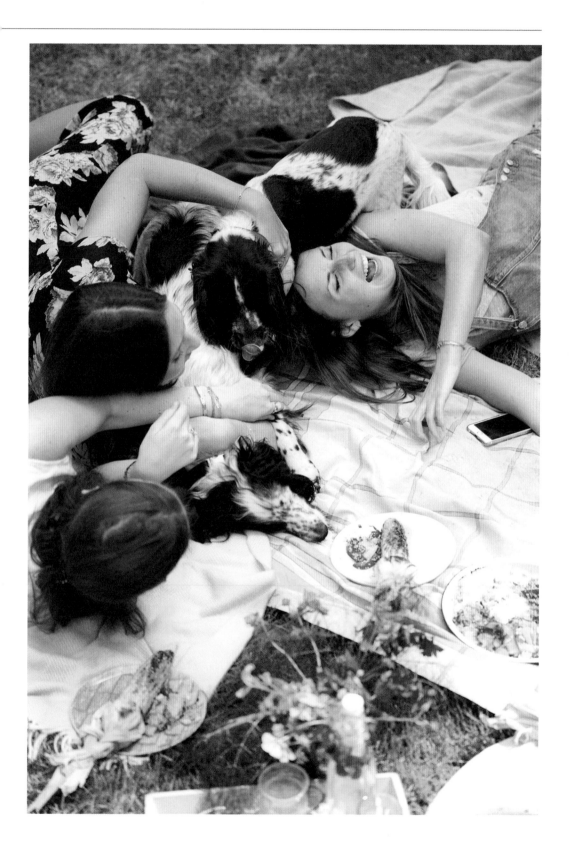

LEMONY POTATO & BUTTER BEAN SALAD

This is the perfect simple salad for a light lunch. It's full of subtle flavours that won't overwhelm your palate, but will make you really happy! The mix of lemony potatoes, soft butter beans and peppery rocket is a winning combination, especially when served with juicy vine tomatoes. I love eating this with my Baked Sesame & Tomato Avocados (page 85), but it also works really well as a side salad, or just on its own with a good dollop of hummus.

Serves 4

NUT-FREE

350g baby potatoes, well scrubbed
salt and pepper
400g can of butter beans,
    drained and rinsed
finely grated zest and juice of
    1 unwaxed lemon
olive oil
1 bag of rocket, or a mix of rocket,
    watercress, spinach
a couple of big vine tomatoes,
    cut into wedges
handful of fresh basil leaves

Put the potatoes into a pan of water, add a little salt, place the lid on and bring it to the boil. Once boiling, reduce the heat to a simmer and cook until you can pass a sharp knife through the middle of the biggest potato. This should take 10–15 minutes.

When cooked, drain the potatoes and put them into a bowl with the butter beans, the lemon zest and juice, salt and pepper and a drizzle of olive oil. Mix together, and set aside to cool.

Put the salad leaves and tomatoes in a big bowl, season the tomatoes very well, then scatter the potatoes and butter beans on top. Drizzle some olive oil over and top with the basil to serve.

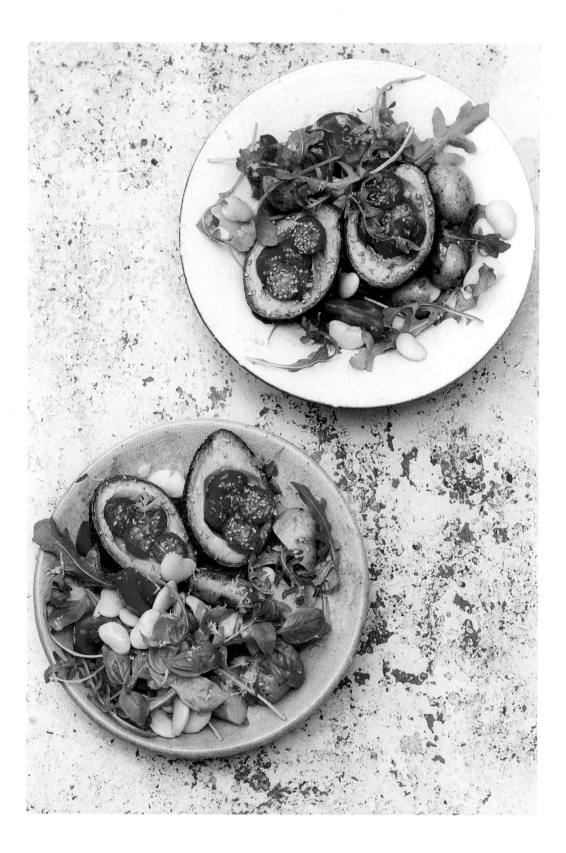

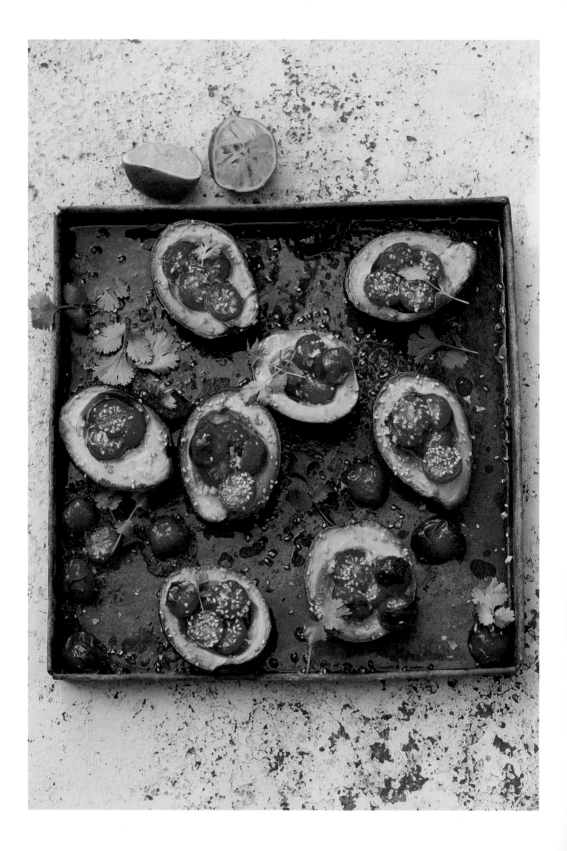

BAKED SESAME & TOMATO AVOCADOS

These taste amazing. If you've never baked an avocado before, you've been missing out!
As the avocado bakes, the tomatoes split open, which makes them extra soft and tender,
while filling them with flavour. They look so beautiful too, with the mix of green and red.
These are a great quick lunch with the Lemony Potato & Butter Bean Salad (page 82),
or with Mango & Mushroom Ceviche (page 66), or as a delicious addition to brunch.

Serves 2 as a main, or 4 with another dish

NUT-FREE

2 ripe avocados

100g cherry tomatoes, plus more if you
    have them

2 garlic cloves, crushed

3 teaspoons toasted sesame oil

olive oil

salt and pepper

4 teaspoons sesame seeds

juice of 2 limes

small handful of fresh coriander, chopped

Preheat the oven to 200°C (fan 180°C).

Halve the avocados and remove the stones.
With a spoon, scoop out a little of the flesh
to make the hole a bit bigger (you don't need
this spare flesh, so now is a good time to
snack on the leftovers).

Cut the tomatoes in half, then mix with the
garlic, 1 teaspoon of the sesame oil, a drizzle
of olive oil and lots of salt and pepper.

Place the avocado halves on to a baking tray,
scrunching up a little foil and resting each
half on top to keep them steady while they're
cooking. Evenly fill them with the tomato mix.

Place any spare tomatoes around the
avocados to bake alongside (they look
particularly beautiful if they're on the vine).

Drizzle everything with a little more olive oil,
sprinkle with salt and pepper, then bake for
15–20 minutes.

Put the baked avocados on to plates, then
sprinkle 1 teaspoon of sesame seeds and
squeeze the juice of ½ lime over each
avocado half, as well as the rest of the
sesame oil. Then scatter over the chopped
coriander and a little extra salt and serve.

SWEET POTATO NOODLES WITH A CREAMY PEANUT SATAY SAUCE

These noodles were quite a revelation to me. They're so much heartier and more filling than courgette noodles, and this satay sauce really brings them to life. It's so incredibly creamy, with subtle hints of chilli and tangy lime. Together they make for the best pick-me-up dinner, healthy but comforting and bursting with flavour. You will need a spiraliser for this recipe.

Serves 2

FOR THE NOODLES

olive oil

1 celery stick, finely chopped

5 garlic cloves, crushed

2.5cm root ginger, finely grated

pinch of salt

250g mushrooms, thinly sliced

2 small sweet potatoes, about 200g each,
    peeled and spiralised

100g baby spinach

FOR THE SAUCE

3 tablespoons crunchy peanut butter
    (or almond butter also works)

70ml almond milk, plus more if needed

1 teaspoon tamari

1 teaspoon chilli flakes

juice of 1 lime

1 tsp honey

a little olive oil, if needed

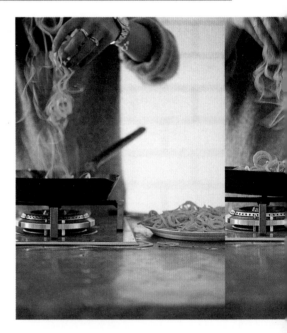

Heat a glug of oil in a large frying pan, then add the celery, garlic, ginger and salt and sauté over a low heat until the celery is softening. Add the mushrooms once the pan has been bubbling for a couple of minutes.

After a minute or so more, add the sweet potatoes and cook for about 10 minutes.

Next, make the satay sauce. Simply place all the ingredients in a blender and blend until smooth, adding oil if it helps to process the sauce, then add salt to taste.

Once the noodles and mushrooms are tender, add the spinach and the satay sauce. Stir until the spinach has wilted and the sauce is warm. If the sauce feels a little thick, add a splash of water, olive oil or almond milk and stir it in until it reaches your desired consistency.

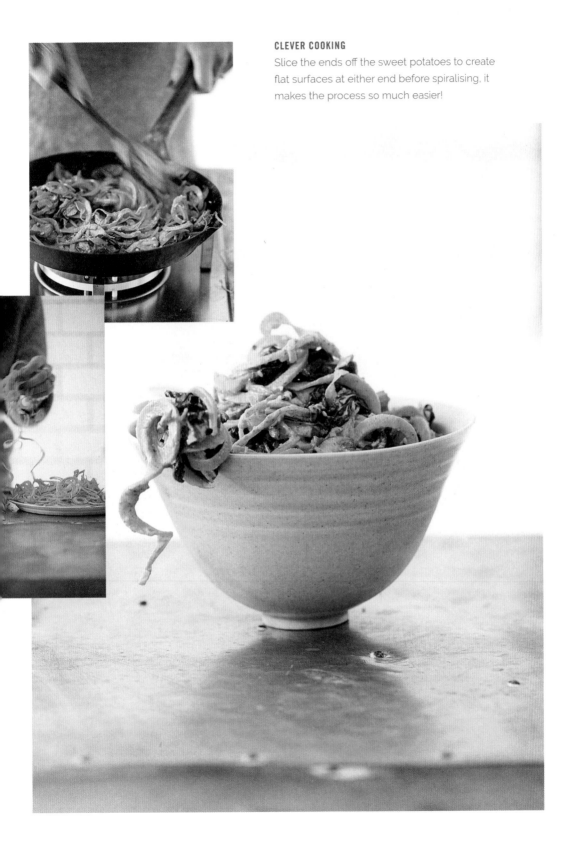

CLEVER COOKING
Slice the ends off the sweet potatoes to create flat surfaces at either end before spiralising, it makes the process so much easier!

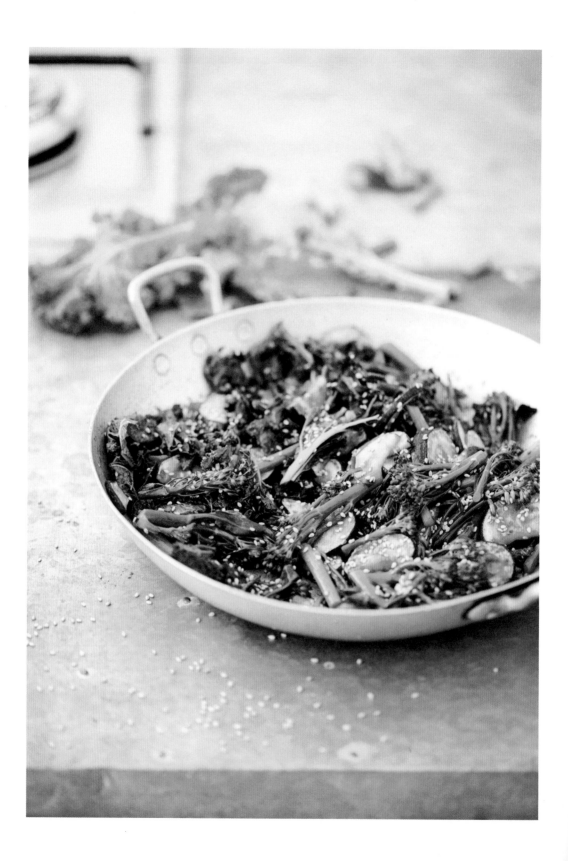

SAUTÉED TAMARI GREENS

These are such a flavoursome but incredibly simple way to add goodness to your meal and work perfectly with the Sweet Potato Noodles with a Creamy Peanut Satay Sauce (page 86). The courgettes, broccoli and kale are lightly sautéed in a mix of tamari and sesame oil; a quick way to transform them into something very delicious!

Serves 4

NUT-FREE

3 tablespoons tamari

2 teaspoons toasted sesame oil

1 tablespoon olive oil

2 courgettes, halved lengthways,
    then cut into half moons

200g Tenderstem broccoli spears,
    each cut into 3

100g torn-up kale, coarse ribs removed

handful of toasted sesame seeds

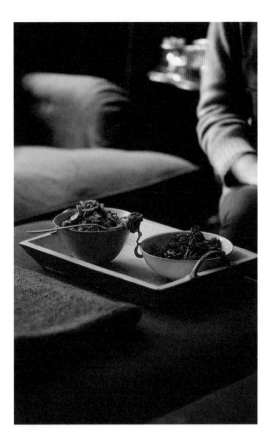

Heat the tamari and oils in a large sauté pan, then add the courgettes and broccoli and stir-fry over a high heat for 3 minutes.

Add the kale and cook for another 2 minutes until the leaves have wilted. Take off the heat and place on a serving plate.

Scatter with the toasted sesame seeds and bring to the table.

PAN TO PLATE

10 minutes

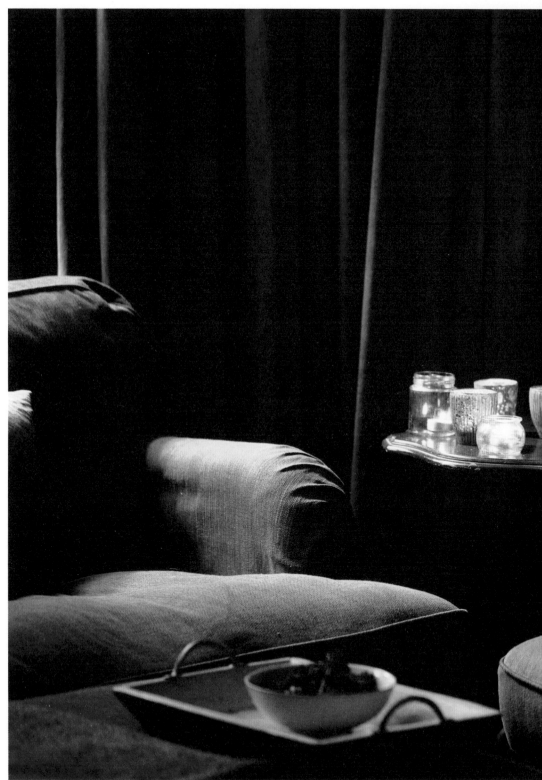

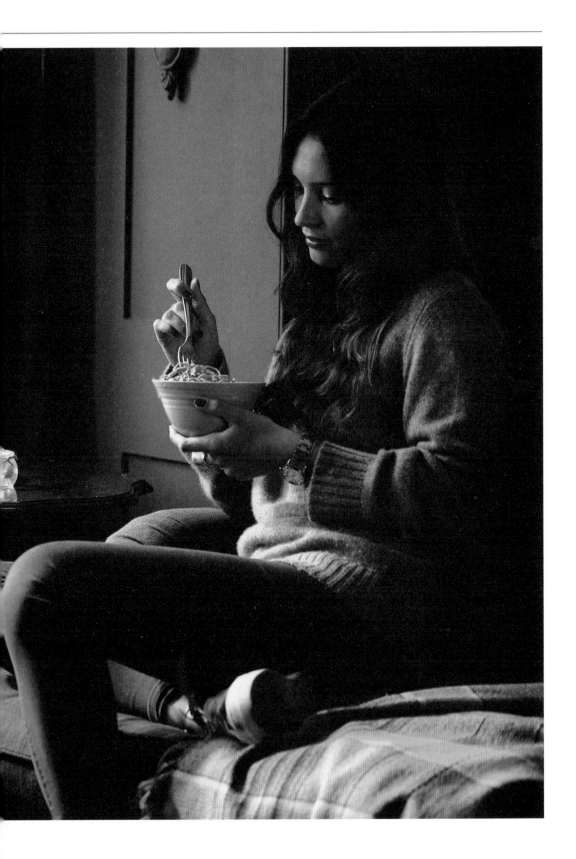

CHILLI & GINGER PHO

This is a simplified version of the classic pho recipe, which means you can have dinner on the table in twenty minutes rather than leaving it to simmer for hours! The broth base is flavoured with sesame, ginger, spring onions, chilli and lime and then filled with lots of veggies and buckwheat noodles before being topped with fresh coriander. A perfect cosy, comforting supper that will warm and rejuvenate you.

Serves 4

NUT-FREE

2 portions of buckwheat noodles,
  or even courgetti
25g dried shiitake mushrooms
2 teaspoons toasted sesame oil
generous thumb of root ginger, finely grated
2 garlic cloves, finely grated
2 red chillies, finely sliced
2 spring onions, each chopped into 4
2 tablespoons brown miso paste
2 tablespoons tamari
100g baby corn
250g bok choi, thinly sliced
120g beansprouts
2 carrots, peeled and julienned
handful of fresh coriander, roughly chopped
juice of 1 lime, plus lime wedges to serve

Prepare the noodles, if using, according to the packet instructions, then place in a sieve and rinse with cold water. Put the dried shiitake in a bowl, pour over 500ml of boiling water and set aside for 20 minutes.

Heat the sesame oil in a wok, or large sauté pan, then add the ginger, garlic, chillies and spring onions, and cook for a minute or so, stirring to make sure the garlic doesn't burn.

Splash in a little water and let it bubble for a couple of minutes, then add the miso and tamari and 500ml more boiling water. Let this broth bubble away until the mushrooms are ready, then add them too, with their soaking water (except the dregs, as they may contain grit). Return to a nice simmer for 5 minutes.

Add the corn and bok choi, and simmer for 5 minutes. Stir in the beansprouts and carrots.

Divide the noodles between 4 bowls, then spoon the broth on top. Sprinkle with chopped coriander and a squeeze of lime juice, then serve with lime wedges.

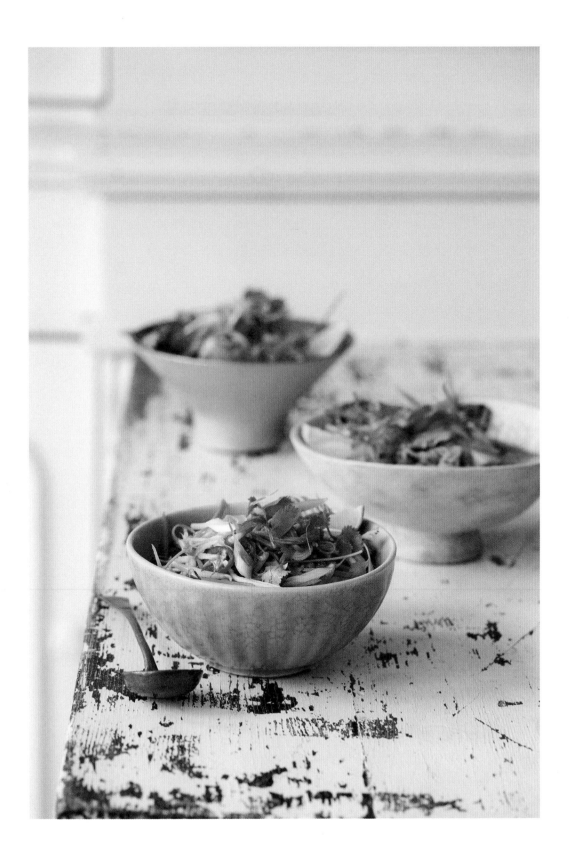

SESAME & MAPLE SUMMER ROLLS WITH SWEET ALMOND DIPPING SAUCE

One of my favourite quick bites. These take just five minutes to make, there's no cooking required and almost no washing-up either, which I love! I serve them to friends when they arrive, as a pre-dinner snack, or use them as a nibble at a party. The flavours work so well with the Chilli & Ginger Pho, too (page 92), it's a perfectly light but incredibly delicious meal.

Makes 10

FOR THE ROLLS

1 cucumber, peeled

small handful of fresh coriander

juice of 1–2 limes (depending how juicy they are; if you don't get much juice from the first, add the second to get a good lime flavour in the dressing)

1 tablespoon maple syrup

1 tablespoon toasted sesame oil

1 tablespoon sesame seeds

1 tablespoon olive oil

salt

10 rice paper wrappers

1 large, ripe avocado, pitted, peeled and chopped

FOR THE DIPPING SAUCE

1 tablespoon almond butter

1 tablespoon sesame seeds

1 tablespoon olive oil

1 tablespoon toasted sesame oil

1 tablespoon maple syrup

juice of 1 lime

1 tablespoon tamari

Chop the cucumber into thin quarter-circles and finely chop the coriander.

Toss the cucumber into a bowl with the lime juice, maple syrup, sesame oil and seeds, coriander, olive oil and salt and let them all sit in the bowl for a few minutes to marinate.

Get the wrappers ready by dipping each into warm water to soften them. Scoop some of the cucumber mix into the middle of each, then add some avocado. Roll the wrapper up. Repeat to make 10 rolls.

Stir all the sauce ingredients together in a bowl, ready for dipping.

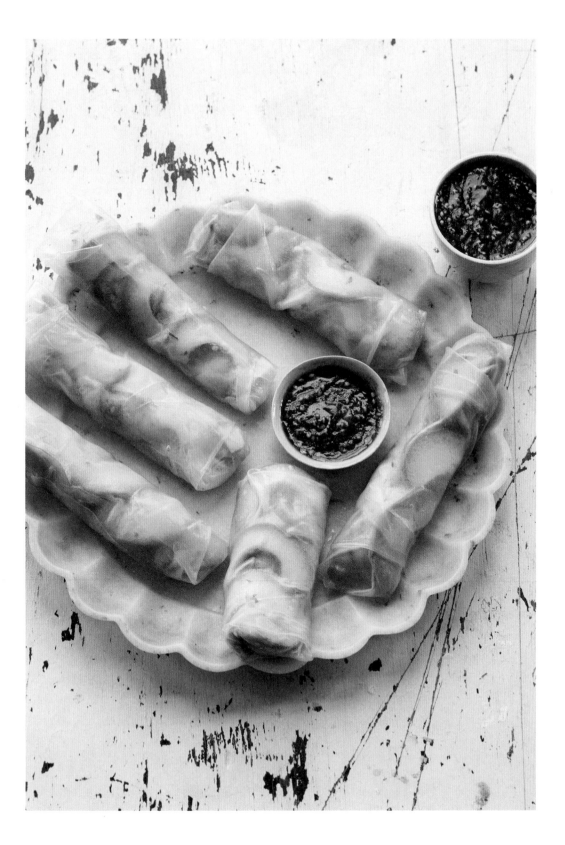

PISTACHIO & APRICOT QUINOA

Wonderfully quick and simple to throw together. This tastes amazing with the soft Asian Sesame Slaw (page 99); together, they're one of my favourite summer lunches. The flavours in this quinoa mixture are wonderfully subtle. The apricots add a lovely sweet, chewy touch, while the bites of cucumber give a freshness and the pistachios create a nutty crunch.

Serves 3

FOR THE QUINOA

200g quinoa

salt

1 small cucumber

15 dried apricots (preferably unsulphured)

80g pistachios

handful of rocket (optional)

FOR THE DRESSING

finely grated zest and juice of
    1 unwaxed lemon

1 teaspoon ground cumin

2 tablespoons apple cider vinegar

4 tablespoons olive oil

salt

Place the quinoa in a saucepan with a generous sprinkling of salt and 500ml of boiling water. Bring to the boil, then let it simmer for 10–15 minutes, or until the water has been absorbed and the quinoa is soft and fluffy. Place in a salad bowl and leave it to cool.

Meanwhile, finely chop the cucumber and cut each apricot into 6.

Mix all the dressing ingredients together.

Mix the cooled quinoa with the cucumber, apricots and most of the pistachios. Then add the dressing and mix it all together.

Finally, sprinkle the remaining pistachios on the top. Serve with rocket, if you like.

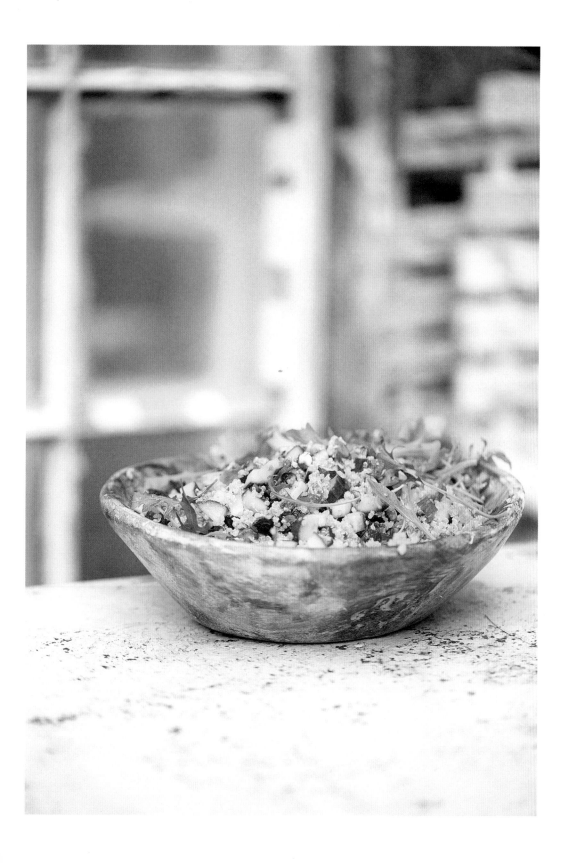

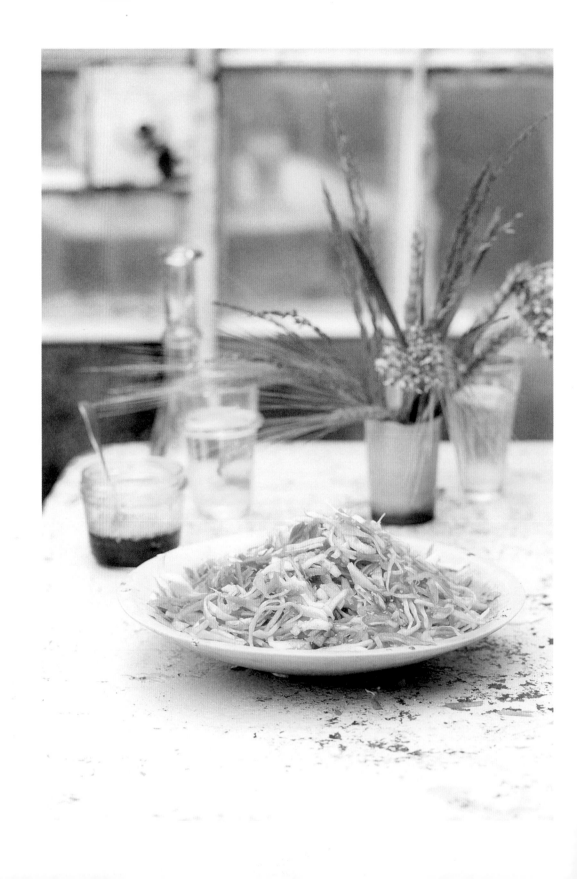

SESAME SLAW

One of my go-to quick salads, this is so easy to make and full of flavour. I know slaw doesn't sound overly exciting — and lots of people wouldn't count cabbage as one of their favourite foods — but this really is so great and so worth trying. I promise you'll be surprised at how much you love it! It tastes amazing with Pistachio & Apricot Quinoa, but I also love it with the Baked Plantains with Sweet Chilli Sauce (pages 96 and 187); they are incredible together.

Serves 3

NUT-FREE

2 carrots

⅓ white cabbage

finely grated zest of 1 unwaxed lime
and juice of 2 limes

2 tablespoons sesame seeds

2 tablespoons toasted sesame oil

5 tablespoons olive oil

2 tablespoons tamari

1 tablespoon honey

generous sprinkling of salt

Start by peeling and grating the carrots (use the fattest holes on the grater, or the grater setting on your food processor). Next, finely shred the cabbage by slicing finely with a sharp knife. Mix together in a bowl.

Zest 1 of the limes, then squeeze the juice of both limes into the bowl and add the grated zest. Add the sesame seeds, sesame oil, olive oil, tamari, honey and salt and stir well, until the carrots and cabbage are totally covered in dressing.

Leave the slaw to sit for 10–20 minutes before serving; this allows it to soften and absorb the flavours of the dressing.

SUPER-SPEEDY
10 minutes, plus marinating time

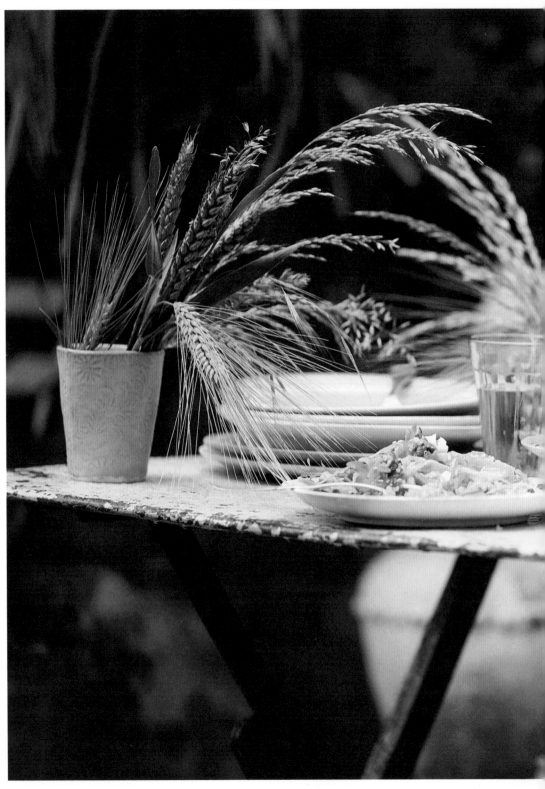

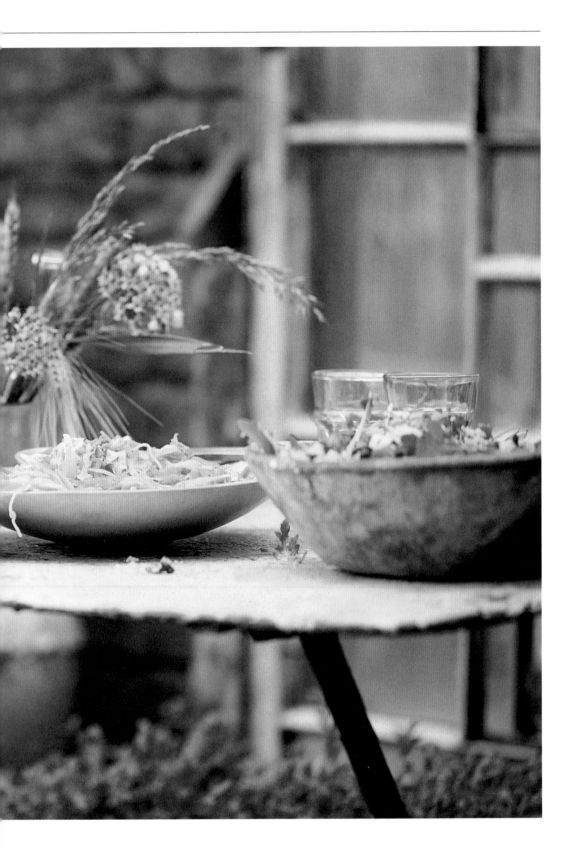

SAUTÉED TEMPEH WITH ROASTED GARLIC & ALMOND PESTO

I've grown to really enjoy tempeh over the last year. It's not overly exciting on its own, but when you sauté it with spring onions and tamari, dunk it into a big bowl of roasted garlic and almond pesto and then scatter it across a Sesame, Coriander & Roasted Fennel Rice Bowl (page 104) it tastes pretty wonderful!

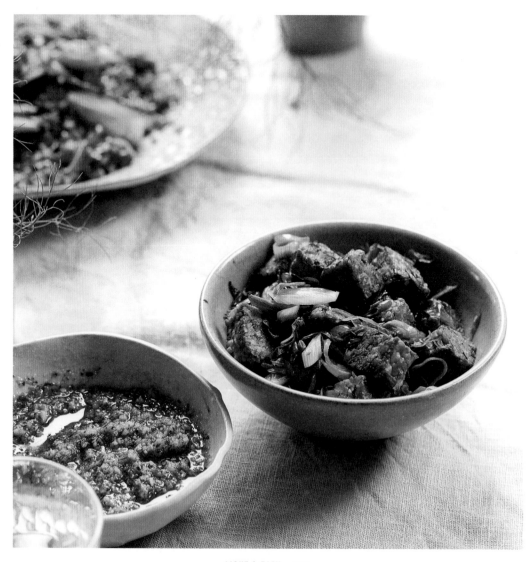

Serves 2

FOR THE PESTO
6 large garlic cloves, unpeeled
100g blanched almonds
50g fresh basil
juice of 1 large lemon
10 tablespoons olive oil
salt

FOR THE TEMPEH
200g tempeh
2 spring onions
2 teaspoons coconut oil
1 teaspoon apple cider vinegar
1 teaspoon tamari

For the pesto, preheat the oven to 200°C (fan 180°C). Place the garlic and almonds on a baking tray and bake for 10 minutes, then remove from the oven and leave to cool.

Once cool, remove the garlic skins, then put the garlic and almonds in a food processor with all the remaining ingredients. Blend until smooth. Scrape into a bowl and set aside.

Cut the tempeh into bite-sized squares and slice the spring onions.

Heat the coconut oil in a frying pan. Once it has melted, add the spring onions, vinegar, tamari and tempeh.

Cook for 10 minutes over a high heat, until the tempeh browns and turns crispy.

Serve the tempeh on top of the Sesame, Coriander & Roasted Fennel Rice Bowl with the pesto. Or add it to any other bowl. I find it's best alongside some quinoa or brown rice.

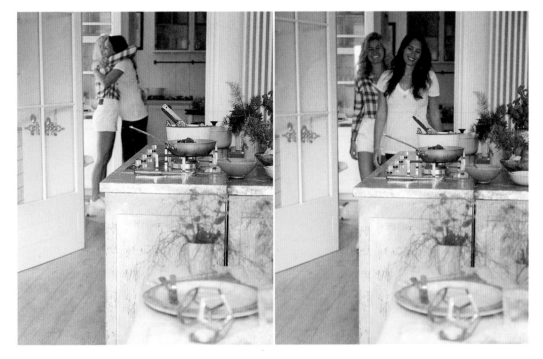

SESAME, CORIANDER & ROASTED FENNEL RICE BOWL

This brown rice bowl with creamy avocado chunks, blackened peppers, roasted fennel and mashed garlic dressing is incredible, one of my absolute best dinners. It's great just on its own, but I also love serving it in bowls with Sautéed Tempeh scattered over the top and a big dollop of creamy Roasted Garlic & Almond Pesto on the side (page 102), which I then dip each bite into for extra flavour!

Serves 2

NUT-FREE

FOR THE RICE BOWL

70g short-grain brown rice

1 tablespoon apple cider vinegar

1 tablespoon tamari

salt

1 fennel bulb

2 red peppers

olive oil

5–10g fresh coriander

1 ripe avocado

2 tablespoons sesame seeds

FOR THE DRESSING

4 garlic cloves, unpeeled

3 tablespoons olive oil

2 teaspoons apple cider vinegar

1 teaspoon tamari

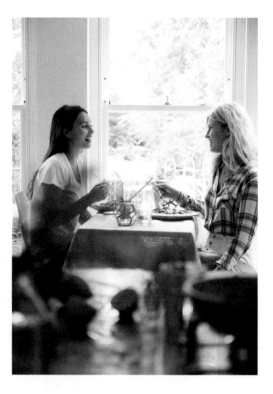

Cook the brown rice with the vinegar, tamari and salt. This should take about 40 minutes.

Preheat the oven to 200°C (fan 180°C).

Cut the fennel lengthways into slices, then cut each pepper into about 8 pieces. Place them on a baking tray, drizzle with olive oil and sprinkle with salt. Bake for 15–20 minutes, until the edges are browning. For the last 10 minutes, add the garlic cloves (they will be used in the dressing).

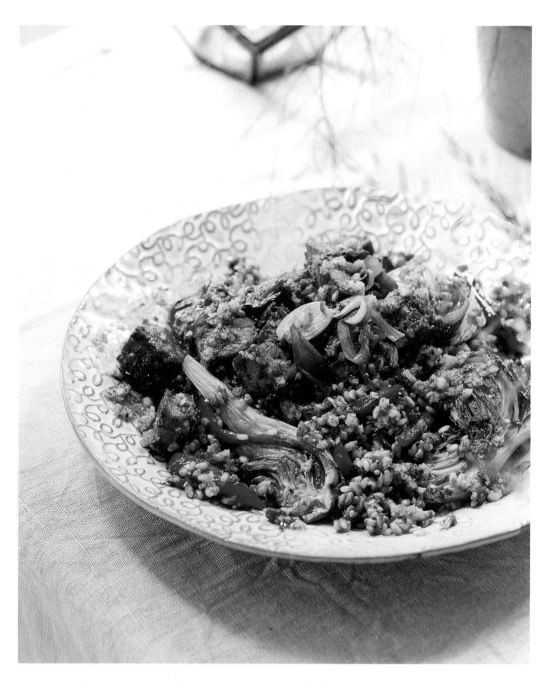

Leave the rice, veg and garlic to cool.

Finely chop the coriander. Peel and pit the avocado and cut it into bite-sized chunks. Roughly chop the roast veg and stir it into the rice, with the sesame seeds and avocado.

Peel the roasted garlic cloves, then mash them with a fork (they should be really soft) and mix with all the other dressing ingredients. Stir into the rice and sprinkle with the coriander. Serve in a beautiful salad bowl.

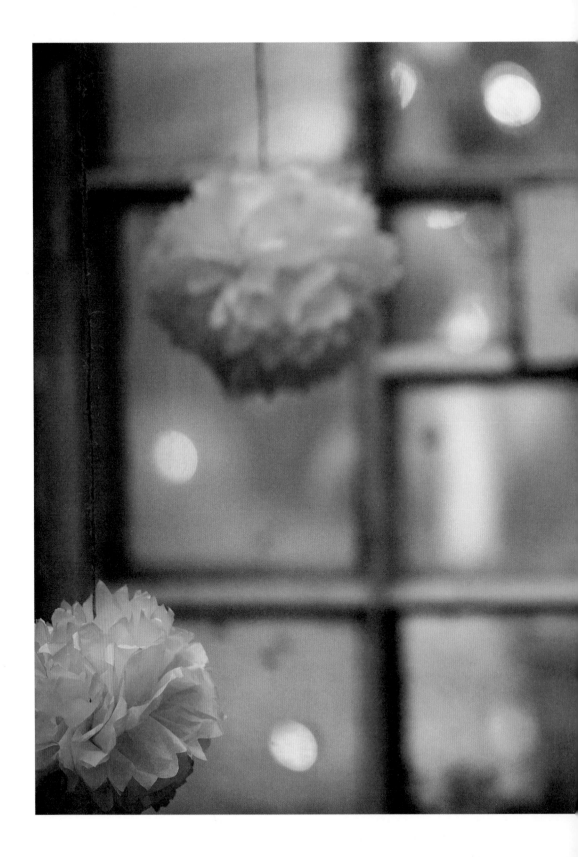

FEASTS

LONG, LAZY DINNERS TO SHARE & SAVOUR

FEASTS

Feasting with friends is one of the best things you can do in life, almost nothing makes me happier than sharing mountains of beautiful food with the people I love most, and that's what this chapter is all about. I hope it will help you find ways to enjoy the kind of food you love with others, so that you can all eat together and they'll see how delicious nutritious food can be. There are so many amazing meals here, but I'm especially keen on bowls of Pea, Courgette & Coconut Risotto served with Chilli Garlic Broccoli for cosy evenings; big platters of Quesadillas with Cashew Sour Cream, &Guacamole, Refried Black Beans & Spicy Salsa for fun nights with friends; and Marinated Cauliflower Steaks with Chilli Quinoa and Sun-dried Tomato & Butter Bean Hummus for summer nights.

MENU

MEXICAN FIESTA

Tortillas for Quesadillas
Refried Black Beans & Spicy Salsa
Cashew Sour Cream & Guacamole

COMFORTING

Pea, Courgette & Coconut Risotto
Chilli Garlic Broccoli

SUNDAY LUNCH

Herbed Nut Roast
Maple Roasted Root Veg
Mushroom Gravy

INDIAN FEAST

Chana Masala
Aloo Gobi
Coconut Rice

GARDEN PARTY

Marinated Cauliflower Steaks with Chilli Quinoa
Sun-dried Tomato & Butter Bean Hummus

COSY KITCHEN SUPPER

Three Bean Stew
Mango Salsa

SIMPLE & INEXPENSIVE

Chickpea Chilli in Baked Sweet Potatoes
Spiced Roast Cauliflower

CURRY NIGHT IN

My Favourite Curried Veggies
Lime & Chilli Pickle

DATE NIGHT

Tomato & Aubergine Bake
Spinach with Mustard Seeds

TORTILLAS FOR QUESADILLAS

This is such a winner; I've always loved quesadillas, so I'm really excited to share this recipe with you. They were my favourite meal at university and I hadn't had them in so long until I created this. Everyone always adores being served one of these beautiful quesadillas stuffed with Refried Black Beans & Spicy Salsa, Cashew Sour Cream & Guacamole (pages 113 and 115). It's a fun meal, and definitely shows people that healthy eating isn't all about kale and carrots… These are best eaten hot and always shared with great friends. They're fun to eat and can get a little messy, so don't make them for a first date!

Makes 8 tortillas / 4 quesadillas

NUT-FREE

200g buckwheat flour
200g polenta
40g milled (ground) chia seeds
2 teaspoons salt
olive oil

Preheat the oven to 200°C (fan 180°C).

Mix all the ingredients except the oil in a bowl, then gradually add 300ml of water, mixing it into a paste with a fork.

On a clean dry surface, lay down a square of baking parchment. Cut another square of parchment and set aside.

Wet your hands and pick up one-eighth of the tortilla mix from the bowl. Roll it in your palms until it's a nice smooth ball and drop it into the centre of the baking parchment. Place the second sheet of baking parchment on top and squash the dough down gently with your hand so it becomes a disc. Take a rolling pin and roll it from the centre outwards to make a circle about 20cm across, then place on a baking sheet. Leave both sheets of baking parchment in place. Repeat with the remaining mix to make 8 tortillas.

Pop them in the oven for 4 minutes. (Do this in batches if you have a small oven.)

As soon as they come out of the oven, peel off all of the baking parchment and set the tortillas aside.

Place a large non-stick frying pan over a high heat. Once it's hot, add a little olive oil, place a tortilla into the pan and load it up with your chosen fillings (pages 113 and 115). Place another tortilla on top, press down to flatten, and cook for 2 minutes. Then flip over gently with a spatula and cook for another 1–2 minutes on the second side. Remove from the heat and cut into quarters or eighths. Repeat the process with the other tortillas.

PAN TO PLATE
20 minutes

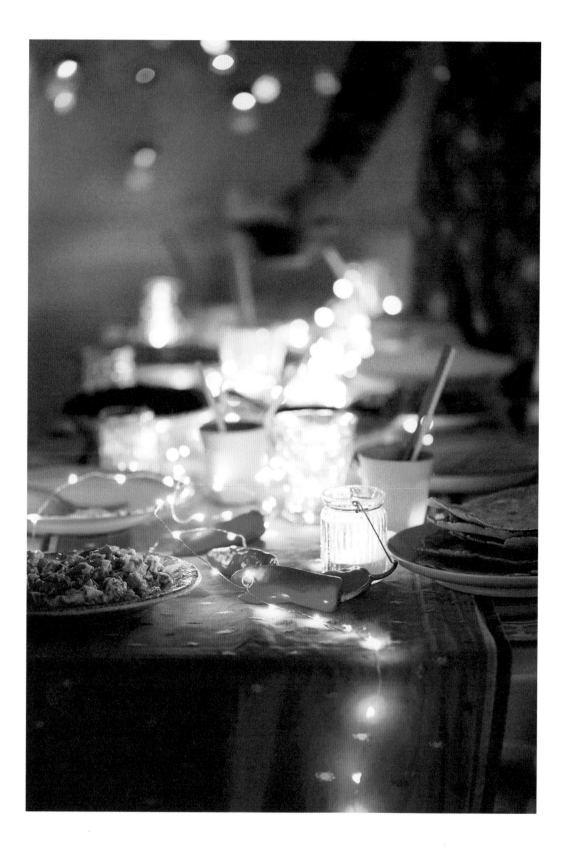

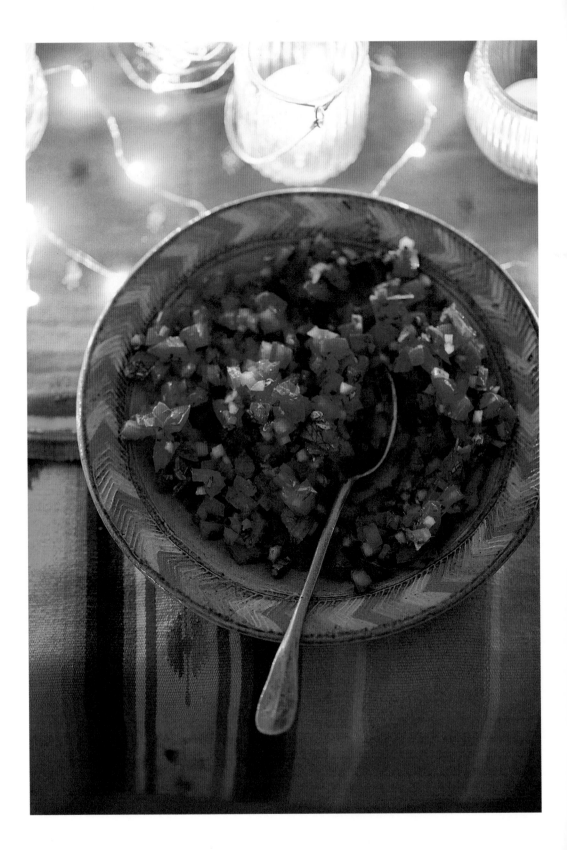

REFRIED BLACK BEANS & SPICY SALSA

These make the most delicious quesadilla filling (page 110). The black beans cook to a comforting, warming mix with a delicious blend of flavours. The tomato salsa brings a slightly spicy and fresher element to the dish, while the beans are heartier with a richer, saltier flavour.

Makes enough for 4 generous quesadillas

NUT-FREE

FOR THE BLACK BEANS

olive oil

4 garlic cloves, crushed

salt and pepper

1 teaspoon ground coriander

½ teaspoon smoked paprika

2 x 400g cans of black beans,
    drained and rinsed

juice of 1 lime

FOR THE SALSA

5 tomatoes, finely chopped

2 red chillies, deseeded and finely chopped

1 tablespoon apple cider vinegar

2 tablespoons olive oil

handful of fresh coriander, chopped

Start by making the black beans. Heat a glug of olive oil in a saucepan, then add the garlic, salt and pepper and fry over a medium heat for about 1 minute until it starts to turn translucent but doesn't colour.

Add the spices, beans and lime juice. Cook for about 10 minutes over a low heat, until the beans start to soften.

Meanwhile, for the salsa, mix everything together in a bowl. Cover and let it sit for at least 5 minutes before eating, so that all the flavours meld together.

Serve in the quesadillas (for how to cook and assemble these, see page 110).

MIX IT UP

I've used 2 chillies in the salsa because I love the spicy heat but, if you prefer, use fewer to your taste.

PAN TO PLATE

15 minutes

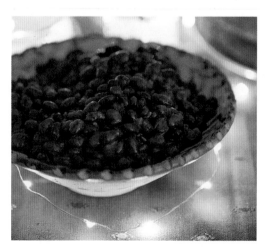

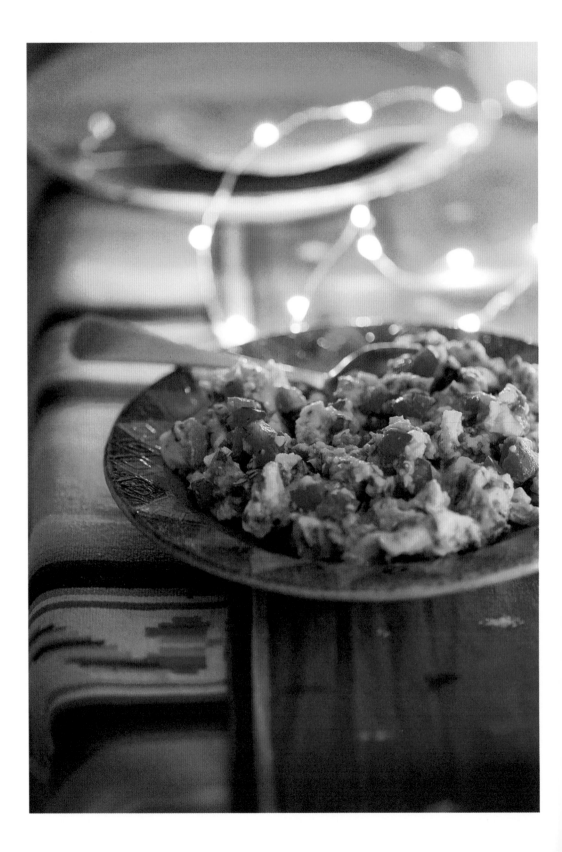

CASHEW SOUR CREAM & GUACAMOLE

These are wonderful additions to quesadillas, as they make each bite so creamy.
I originally made the cashew sour cream for my Mini Baked Potatoes (page 210),
but it was so good I decided I definitely needed to use it in the quesadillas, too! It has a
beautifully smooth texture with wonderful flavours from the chives, vinegar and lemon
juice, plus I find it works perfectly in quesadillas with this chunky guacamole. Remember
that you need to allow soaking time, for the cashews.

Makes 1 big bowl of each, enough for
4 quesadillas

FOR THE CASHEW SOUR CREAM
120g cashew nuts
juice of 1½ lemons
salt and pepper
1 tablespoon apple cider vinegar
5g chives, chopped
3 spring onions, finely chopped

FOR THE GUACAMOLE
3 avocados
juice of 2 limes
1 chilli, deseeded and finely chopped
1 ripe tomato, deseeded and finely chopped
handful of fresh coriander, finely chopped

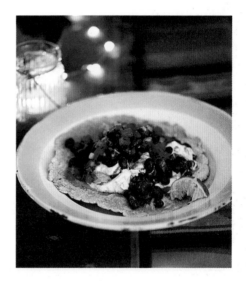

Start the cashew sour cream ahead of time:
put the cashew nuts in a bowl, cover with
water and leave to soak for 4 hours.

Drain the cashew nuts and place them into a
strong blender. Add 2 tablespoons of water,
the lemon juice, salt and pepper and vinegar.
Blend until creamy; this should take a few
minutes. Add the chives and spring onions
and blend for a few seconds, so they are
broken down but not blended smooth. If
you'd like a thinner consistency, add a little
more water.

For the guacamole, pit and peel the
avocados and scoop out the flesh, placing it
into a bowl. Mash with a fork.

Mix all the remaining ingredients with the
mashed avocados and season well.

To assemble the quesadillas, see page 110.

SUPER SPEEDY
10 minutes, plus soaking time

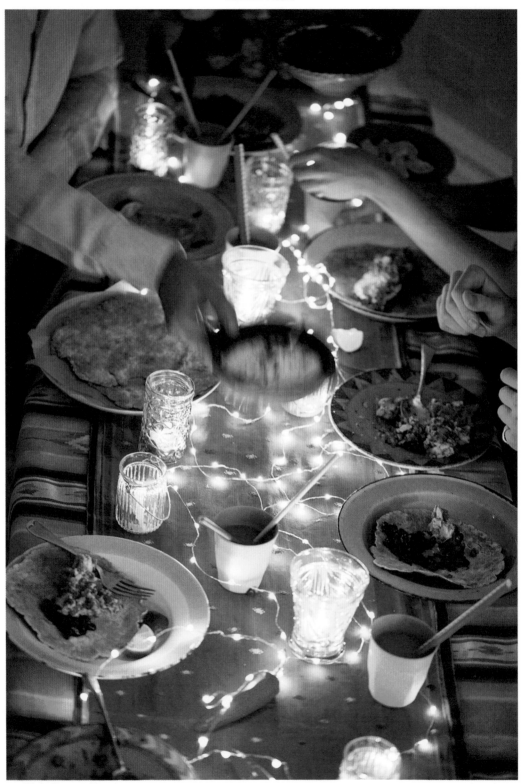

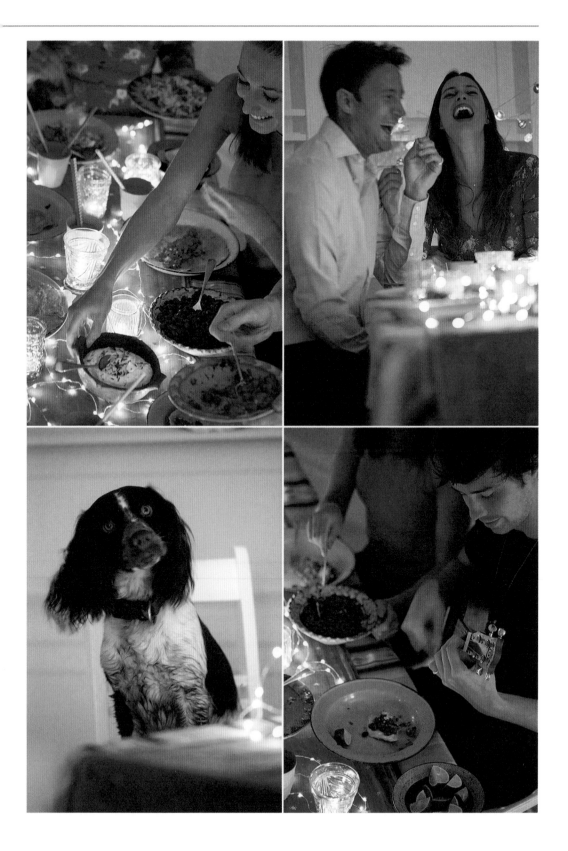

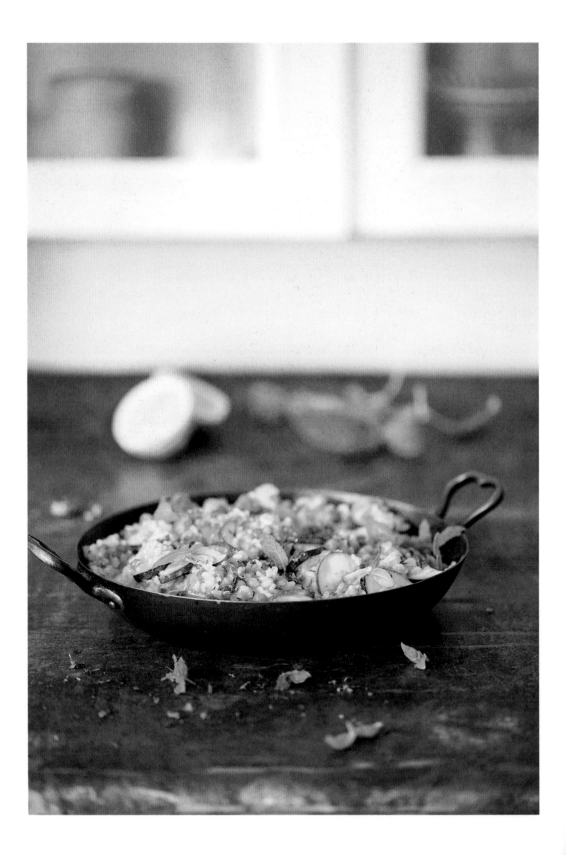

PEA, COURGETTE & COCONUT RISOTTO

This is an absolute dream. It's so wonderfully creamy and flavoursome, yet still light and refreshing. I cook the rice in coconut milk to give it a more traditional risotto texture, then stir in a creamy blend of puréed peas with lemon juice and olive oil to give the finished dish extra flavour and thickness. The first time I made this I shared it with my sister – who's a risotto addict – and she said that she didn't even need to add Parmesan cheese… which was the ultimate compliment from her!

Serves 4

NUT-FREE

FOR THE RISOTTO

olive oil

2 celery sticks, finely chopped

salt and pepper

5 garlic cloves, crushed

350g short-grain brown rice

400ml can of coconut milk

2 tablespoons apple cider vinegar

juice of 1 lemon

2 small courgettes, sliced into half moons

300g frozen peas, defrosted

a few sprigs of fresh mint, leaves picked
    and roughly chopped

FOR THE CREAMY PEA MIX

200g frozen peas, defrosted

juice of 2 lemons

leaves from 20g fresh basil

2 tablespoons nutritional yeast

70ml olive oil

Put a big glug of olive oil in a large saucepan with a lid and set it over a medium heat. Add the celery, salt and pepper and cook for about 10 minutes or until soft. Add the garlic and cook for another minute before adding the rice, coconut milk, 1.2 litres of water, the vinegar and lemon juice. Bring to a boil, then reduce the heat and let it simmer for 50 minutes with the lid on until the rice is cooked and the water is absorbed. Check it every now and again and give it a stir. You may need to add slightly more water during cooking, as the water can be absorbed at different speeds depending on the shape of your pan and the heat under it.

When the 50 minutes is up, take the lid off the risotto, add the courgettes, stir through and cook for 5 minutes. Throw in the 300g of defrosted peas and stir through again, cook for another 5 minutes, then take off the heat.

While the courgette and peas are warming in the risotto, make the pea mix; simply place all the ingredients into a blender, season well and blend until smooth.

Stir the creamy pea mix through the risotto, sprinkle with the chopped mint and serve.

CHILLI GARLIC BROCCOLI

This is a wonderfully simple side that goes with absolutely everything. I find it especially good with the Pea, Courgette & Coconut Risotto though (page 119). I love the contrast of the slightly crunchy broccoli and the soft, creamy risotto. It's a lovely way to up the amount of greens in any meal, while adding more flavour and extra texture.
I normally use at least six cloves of sautéed garlic in this as I like the flavour to be really strong and come through in every bite, but feel free to tone it down if you want something equally delicious but more subtle.

Serves 4 as a side dish

NUT-FREE

good glug of olive oil

salt and pepper

4–6 garlic cloves, crushed

1 red chilli, deseeded and finely chopped

400g Tenderstem broccoli

juice of ½ lemon

Heat the olive oil in a wok or a large saucepan with the salt and pepper, garlic and chilli. Let this cook over a medium heat for about 3 minutes until the garlic has softened but not coloured.

Meanwhile, trim the ends from the broccoli, then cut each spear into 3.

Add the broccoli to the pan, increase the heat, add the lemon juice and – while keeping it moving using a wooden spoon – cook for about 5 minutes, until it's tender on the outside but still with a little bite.

PAN TO PLATE

10 minutes

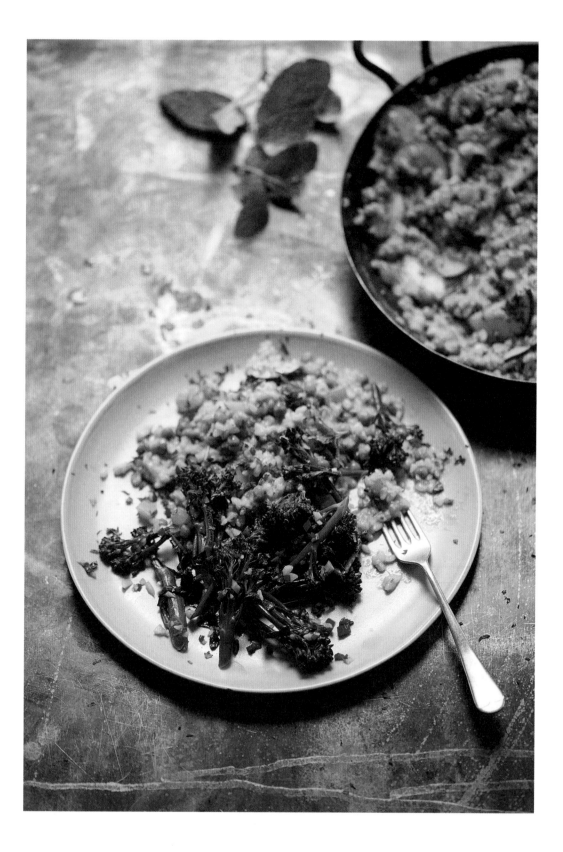

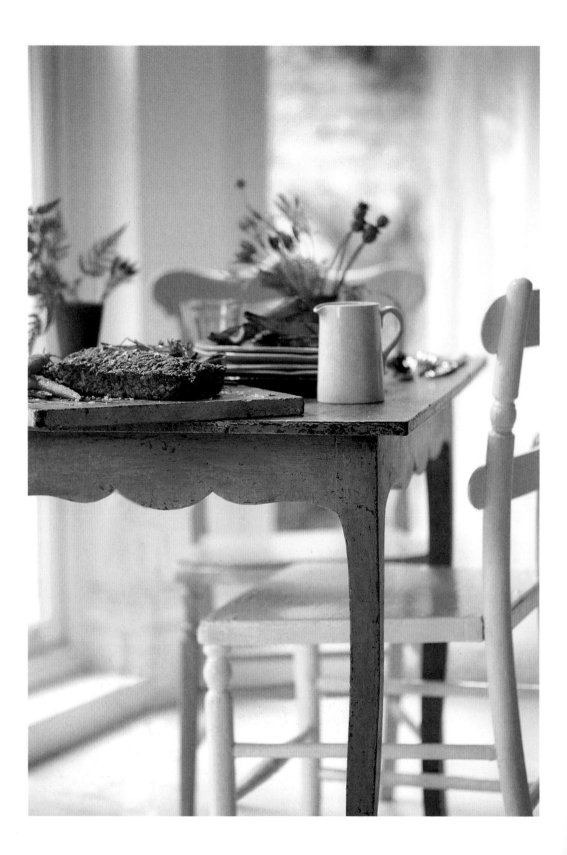

HERBED NUT ROAST

*The ideal veggie option to share with friends for a long, lazy Sunday lunch. It's lovely
and hearty and full of flavour from the pine nuts and cashews to the nutmeg, garlic, sage,
tarragon, garlic and parsley. I love this with a pile of Maple Roasted Root Veg and a big
spoonful of Smashed Turmeric & Mustard Seed Potatoes (pages 126 and 180).*

Serves 6

2 tablespoons olive oil, plus more for the tin

50g pine nuts

75g cashews

1 celery stick, finely chopped

200g butternut squash, peeled and
    finely chopped

1 medium carrot, peeled and finely chopped

salt and pepper

3 garlic cloves, crushed

150g chestnut mushrooms, finely chopped

2 fresh sage leaves, roughly chopped

1 tablespoon roughly chopped
    fresh parsley

1 tablespoon roughly chopped
    fresh tarragon

good few gratings of nutmeg

25g oats

75g brown rice flour

½ tbsp milled (ground) chia seeds

CLEVER COOKING

You need roughly the top part of a butternut
squash for this (the bit from the stalk to the
bulge), so save the rest for later or use it as a
side, roasted or mashed. Also, you can roast
the squash seeds with a drizzle of oil and
seasoning for 10 minutes, then sprinkle them
over sautéed greens.

Preheat the oven to 200°C (fan 180°C). Oil
a 23cm-long loaf tin, or line it with baking
parchment. Place the pine nuts and cashews
on a baking tray and toast them in the oven
for about 10 minutes. They should look
golden and give off a toasty aroma when you
take them out. Set aside to cool.

Meanwhile, place a large non-stick pan over
a medium heat and heat the 2 tablespoons
of oil. Sauté the celery, squash and carrot in
the oil with lots of salt and pepper. When the
celery has started to turn translucent, add the
garlic for 1 minute, then add the mushrooms
and cook for 5 minutes. Finally, add the herbs
and nutmeg and stir well.

Place half the nuts in a food processor with
the oats and whizz up as fine as they will go.
Coarsely chop the remaining nuts, so they
aren't too chunky, then add these and the
ground nut mixture to the pan. Add the flour
and chia seeds and mix well.

Press into the prepared tin, cover with foil
and roast for 35 minutes. Take the foil off and
cook for another 15 minutes. Remove from
the oven and leave, in the tin, on a cooling
rack, for 15 minutes (it will still be nice and
hot). Take it out of the tin and cut into slices;
be gentle, as it can crumble. Serve with
Mushroom Gravy (page 126).

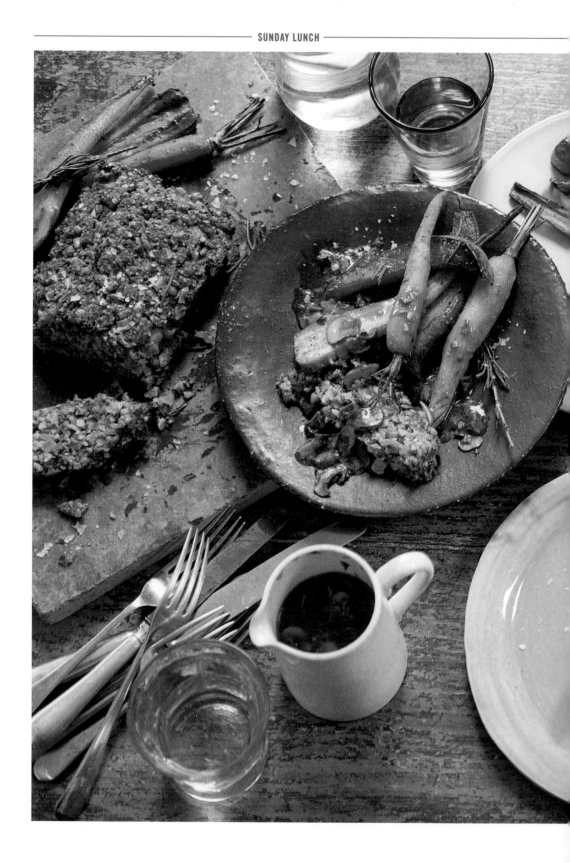

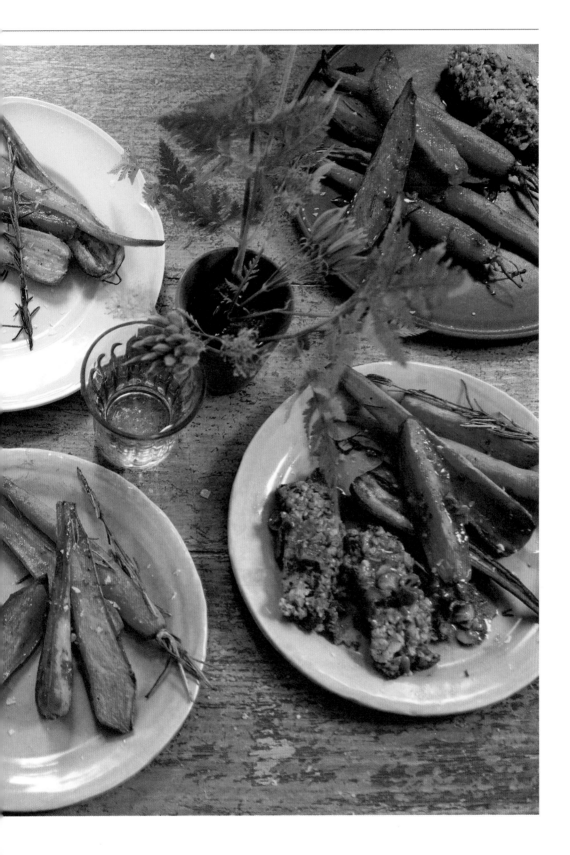

MAPLE ROASTED ROOT VEG

A really simple recipe, but the best addition to your Sunday lunch. Maple syrup brings out the natural sweetness of the veggies, while the paprika, cayenne and rosemary add a whole new level of flavour. The veg become so sweet and tender when baked like this, so everyone will love them! If you're not ready to go full veggie and serve these with a nut loaf, then try adding them to a conventional roast instead; it's a great way to start getting your friends and family excited about plant-based meals.

Serves 4–6

NUT-FREE
2 sweet potatoes, scrubbed well
4 carrots, peeled
4 parsnips, peeled
olive oil
3 tablespoons maple syrup
1 teaspoon smoked paprika
½ teaspoon cayenne pepper
6 sprigs of fresh rosemary
salt and pepper

Preheat the oven to 200°C (fan 180°C).

Cut the sweet potatoes into equal-sized wedges and halve the carrots and parsnips lengthways. Place in a large baking tray in a single layer, or spread them over 2 trays. Drizzle with olive oil and maple syrup, then sprinkle the paprika and cayenne over. Toss everything together, then tuck the rosemary into the veg and season to taste.

Roast for 60 minutes, turning once or twice in that time. When they're finished cooking, the veg should be golden and sticky, with edges that are slightly crisp… delicious!

MUSHROOM GRAVY

The mushrooms and tamari give deeply savoury flavours to this gravy. Sharpened with a little mustard and made aromatic with tarragon, it makes Sunday lunch a real treat. If you like lots of gravy, double the quantities here.

Makes enough for the nut roast

10g dried porcini mushrooms
2 tablespoons rapeseed oil, more if needed
150g chestnut mushrooms, thinly sliced
2 garlic cloves, crushed

salt and pepper
1 tablespoon finely chopped fresh tarragon
1 teaspoon Dijon mustard
1 tablespoon cornflour
1 tablespoon tamari

Put the dried porcini in a bowl with 500ml of boiling water and soak for at least 10 minutes.

Heat the oil in a non-stick frying pan over a high heat. Add the fresh mushrooms and let them colour on both sides, then reduce the heat to low, add the garlic and season. (If the pan is dry, add a bit more oil.) Keep the garlic moving so it doesn't brown, or it will be bitter. Remove the porcini from their water, finely chop and add to the pan, reserving the water.

Once the garlic is translucent, add the tarragon, 400ml of the mushroom water (avoiding any grit from the bottom of the bowl) and the mustard. Mix the cornflour with 1 tablespoon of water to a paste, add to the pan and let simmer for 5–10 minutes until it has a nice consistency. Add the tamari. Serve with the nut roast.

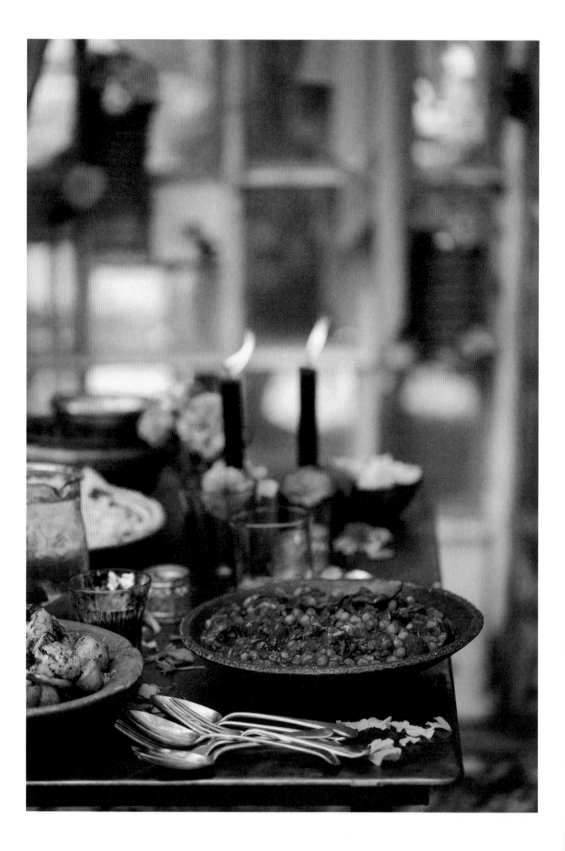

CHANA MASALA

Absolutely delicious and filled with incredible spices that really transform the chickpeas. I also add leeks and spinach, as I love getting the extra veg in and they add a great flavour, plus the green of the spinach makes the meal look beautiful, too. I love this served alongside my Aloo Gobi and Coconut Rice (pages 130 and 133), with a generous dollop of coconut yogurt.

Serves 6

NUT-FREE

5 tablespoons olive oil

6 curry leaves, or 1 teaspoon curry powder

1 leek, finely chopped

½ teaspoon ground turmeric

2 tablespoons ground cumin

2 tablespoons ground coriander

2 tablespoons garam masala

1 teaspoon chilli powder

1 onion, finely chopped

2.5cm root ginger, finely grated

5 garlic cloves, finely grated

2 x 400g cans of chopped tomatoes

2 tablespoons tomato purée

2 green finger chillies, halved lengthways

plenty of salt and pepper

2 x 400g cans of chickpeas,
    drained and rinsed

250g baby leaf spinach

juice of ½ lemon

fresh coriander leaves, to serve

CLEVER COOKING

Make extra so that you have leftovers. As with most curries, this tastes even better the next day, as the flavours have had a chance to develop further, so it's worth saving some to enjoy in your lunch box!

Heat the oil in a large saucepan and throw in the curry leaves, if using. Let them sizzle away and release their flavour for a few minutes, then drop in the leek and stir.

Next add the dry spices – including the curry powder if you're not using curry leaves – and stir so that they're mixed nicely with the leek. Let this cook for a few minutes before adding the onion, ginger and garlic; at this point you can add 1–2 tablespoons of water if things are starting to stick to the pan. Cook for a few minutes before adding the canned tomatoes, tomato purée, green chillies, salt and pepper. When you've poured in the tomatoes from their cans, swish a little water around in each to get the remaining juice, then add this to the saucepan, too. Let everything bubble away for 20 minutes.

Add the chickpeas and cook for another 10 minutes.

Stir in the spinach, just until it wilts. Let cool slightly, then stir in the lemon juice and serve in shallow bowls, sprinkling coriander leaves over the curry.

ALOO GOBI

Matt and I have a favourite little Indian restaurant near our flat that we go to all the time, and I always get the aloo gobi and chana masala. I think the two taste so great together and when I make them at home I serve them on a bed of creamy Coconut Rice (page 133), which makes the meal even better. I love the mix of flavours, that transform the cauliflower and potato into something very special that I hope you'll all really enjoy.

Serves 6

NUT-FREE

2 small cauliflowers, broken into florets
4 tablespoons olive oil
salt and pepper
500g baby potatoes, well scrubbed, quartered
½ cinnamon stick
½ teaspoon whole black peppercorns
5 green cardamom pods, bashed
1 tablespoon mustard seeds
½ teaspoon ground turmeric
2 teaspoons ground cumin
2 teaspoons ground coriander
5 garlic cloves, finely grated
2.5cm root ginger, finely grated
100g cherry tomatoes, halved
2 tablespoons tomato purée
1 tablespoon apple cider vinegar
2 green finger chillies, sliced
juice of ½ lemon
fresh coriander leaves, chopped, to serve

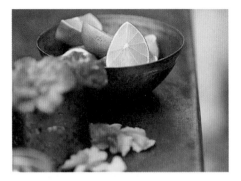

Preheat the oven to 220°C (fan 200°C).

Place the cauliflower in a large baking tray, drizzle with a little of the oil, sprinkle with salt and place into the hot oven for 20 minutes, giving it a shake halfway through cooking.

Meanwhile, boil the potatoes for 10–15 minutes or until cooked through. Once cooked, drain and set aside.

In a large saucepan, gently heat the remaining olive oil, then add all the dry spices. Cook for a few minutes, stirring every now and again, until you start to smell the aromas being released.

Now add the garlic, ginger, tomatoes, tomato purée, vinegar and green chillies, pour in 200ml of water and cook for about 3 minutes, then add the cooked potatoes and cauliflower, squeeze on the lemon juice, season generously with salt and pepper and stir so that all the vegetables are coated in the spiced sauce.

Cook for 5 minutes, then it's ready to eat.

Sprinkle with the fresh coriander and eat with Chana Masala and Coconut Rice (pages 129 and 133).

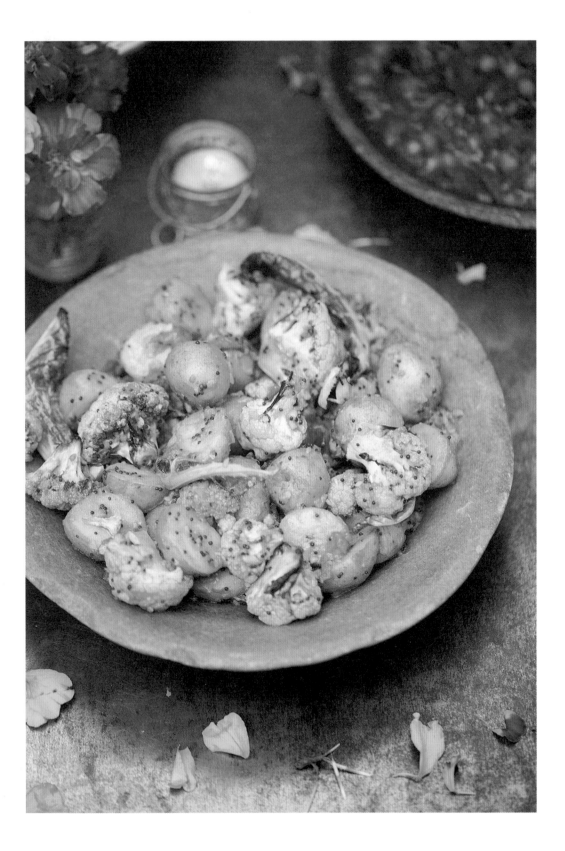

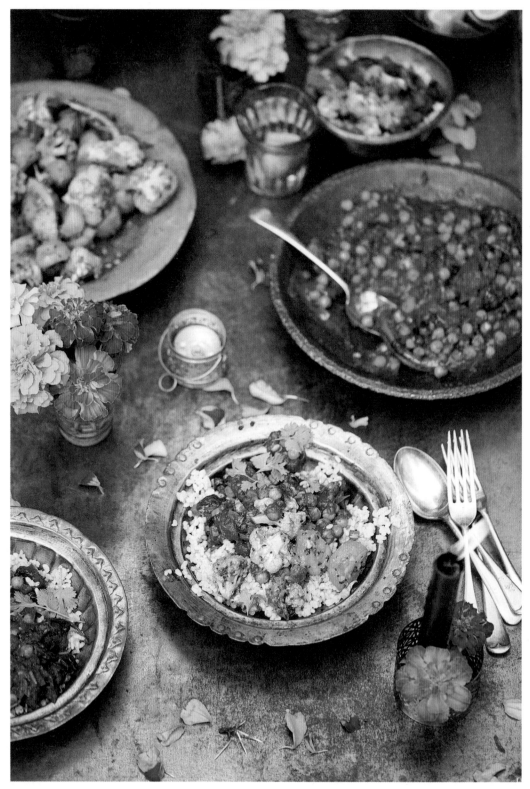

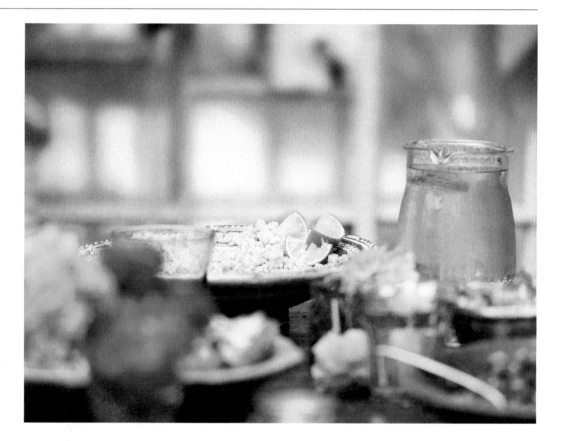

COCONUT RICE

I first ate coconut rice on a trip to Colombia a few years ago and really fell in love with it; it's the best way to make humble rice into something really fabulous. I think it makes the perfect base for your Indian-inspired feast, as it's subtle and simple, which means it's able to soak up all the incredible flavours and spices of the Aloo Gobi and Chana Masala (pages 130 and 129), while adding its own creamy element to each bite.

Serves 6

NUT-FREE

500g short-grain brown rice
400ml can of coconut milk
juice of 2 limes
generous sprinkling of salt

Put the rice into a pan. Add the coconut milk, lime juice, salt and 800ml of boiling water. Stir well and cover the pan.

Bring to the boil, then reduce the heat to a simmer and cook for about 45 minutes, or until perfectly cooked.

CLEVER COOKING

Try making your rice like this to serve with all your stews and curries, your friends will love it!

MARINATED CAULIFLOWER STEAKS WITH CHILLI QUINOA

This dish is just bursting with flavour. The cauliflower steaks are marinated for an hour in a beautiful mix of spices and lemon juice, then baked to create something really special. I serve them on a bed of avocado- and spinach-filled quinoa infused with fresh coriander, sesame oil and tamari. It all sounds, looks and tastes so impressive, but don't worry, it's actually a really easy meal to pull off! Make sure you add Sun-dried Tomato & Butter Bean Hummus on the side (page 137), as it really finishes the dish off perfectly.

Serves 4

NUT-FREE

FOR THE CAULIFLOWER STEAKS

2 cauliflower heads, cut into 4 thick 'steaks'

½ teaspoon ground turmeric

2 teaspoons ground cumin

2 teaspoons paprika

½ teaspoon chilli powder

50ml olive oil

salt and pepper

juice of ½ lemon

FOR THE CHILLI QUINOA

200g quinoa

20g fresh coriander, finely chopped

1 red chilli, deseeded and finely chopped

1 avocado

3 tablespoons olive oil

2 tablespoons apple cider vinegar

juice of ½ lemon

1 tablespoon toasted sesame oil

1 tablespoon tamari

½ teaspoon chilli powder

100g spinach

Place the cauliflower steaks in a single layer on a large baking tray. Whisk all the remaining cauliflower ingredients together in a bowl, with 25ml of water, to make a dressing. Pour this over the cauliflower and turn to make sure each steak is evenly coated. Leave to marinate for at least 1 hour.

Preheat the oven to 180°C (fan 160°C). Roast for about 40 minutes until tender, turning every so often.

Meanwhile, make the quinoa. Place the quinoa into a saucepan with 450ml of water and a little salt. Place the lid on, bring it to the boil, then reduce the heat to a simmer; it should take 12–15 minutes to cook.

Mix the coriander and chilli. Peel and pit the avocado, mash the flesh, then mix it with the coriander and chilli, the olive oil, vinegar, lemon juice, sesame oil and tamari. Season well and stir in the chilli powder. Once the quinoa is cooked, stir in the spinach so that it wilts a little, then stir in the avocado mixture.

Place each cauliflower steak on a bed of quinoa and add a big dollop of Sun-dried Tomato & Butter Bean Hummus (page 137).

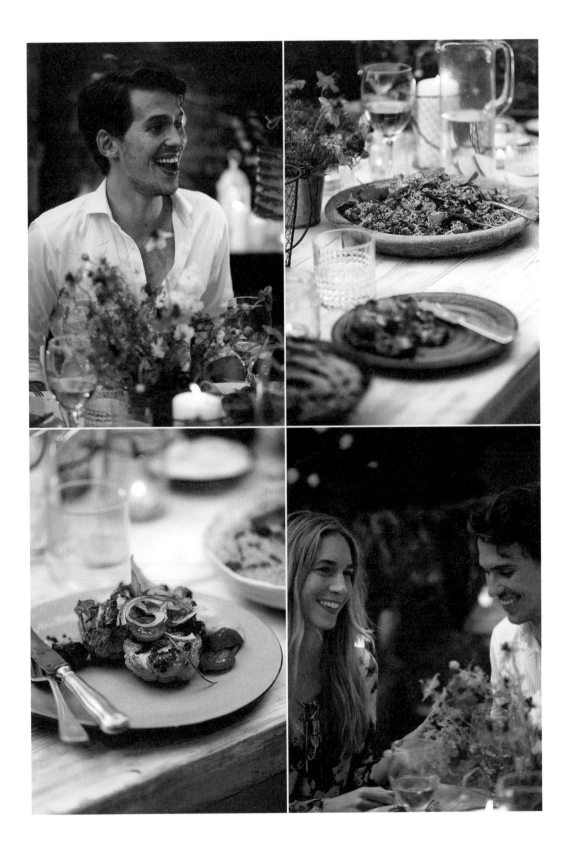

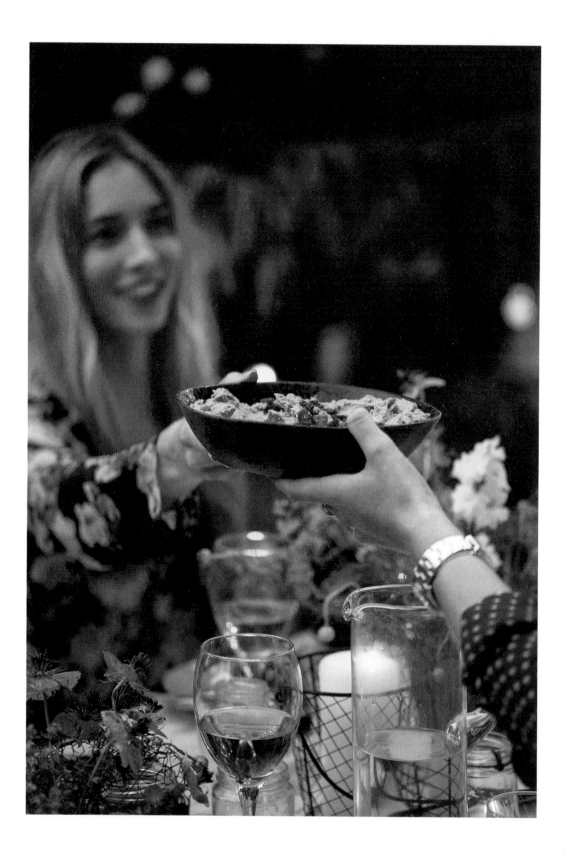

SUN-DRIED TOMATO & BUTTER BEAN HUMMUS

As many of you might know by now, I am a hummus addict: it's my all-time favourite food and something I eat pretty much every day. As a result I'm always looking for new and improved ways to make it, and this version is incredible. It's a great dish for sharing with friends, too, I normally have a bowl ready and waiting for them when they arrive for dinner. The butter beans make the hummus especially creamy, while the sun-dried tomatoes add a wonderfully rich flavour. This tastes absolutely delicious with the Marinated Cauliflower Steaks (page 134) as it really complements the mix of spices in that dish, but it also tastes amazing with simple crackers and crudités as a snack. I normally make extra, so I can keep a bowl in the fridge and enjoy it all week.

Makes a very large bowlful

NUT-FREE

2 x 400g cans of butter beans,
   drained and rinsed
280g jar of sun-dried tomatoes in oil,
   drained (170g drained weight)
2 tablespoons tahini
juice of 2 lemons
2 teaspoons ground cumin
2 tablespoons olive oil
½ tablespoon apple cider vinegar
salt and pepper

Simply place all the ingredients into a food processer with 50ml of water and blend until smooth and creamy. Season to taste.

Store any leftovers in an airtight jar in the fridge; they will keep well for 5–7 days.

SUPER SPEEDY
10 minutes

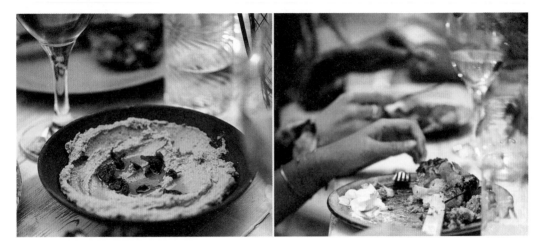

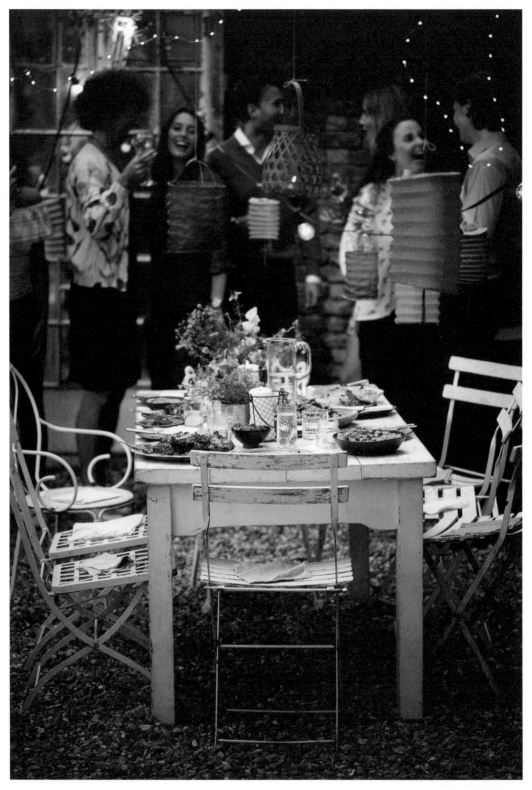

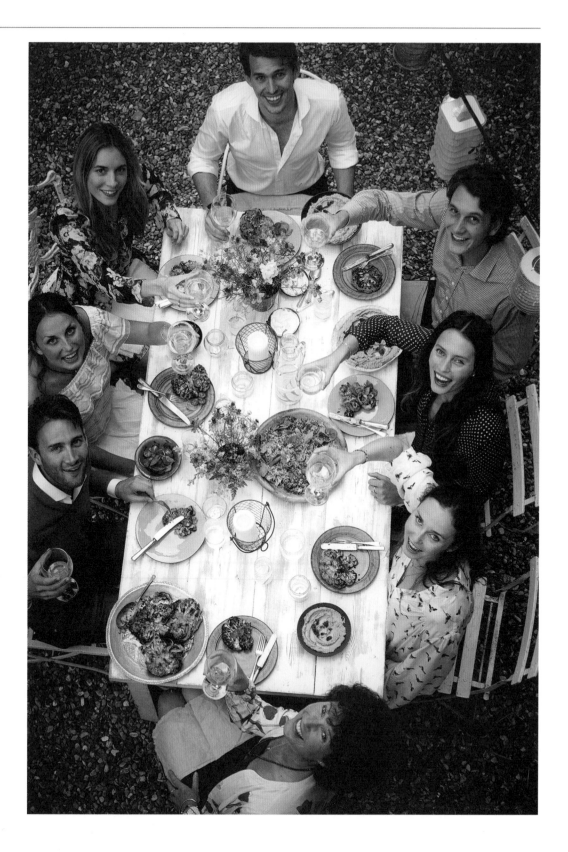

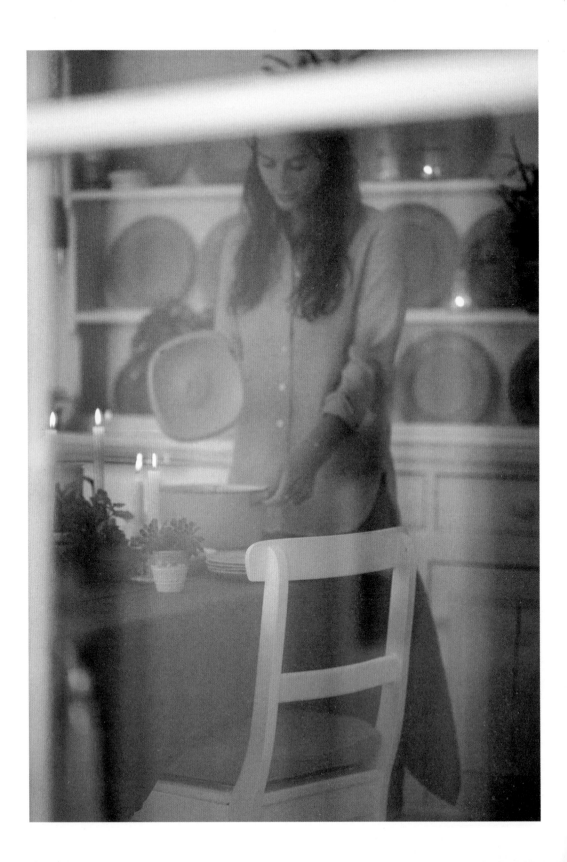

THREE BEAN STEW

As soon as autumn arrives and the weather cools down, I start making this all the time. It's a warming, hearty dish that tastes lovely served on a hot bed of brown rice or quinoa with a big dollop of Mango Salsa on top (page 143). I love the mix of black, butter and cannellini beans; they create such a fantastic mix of textures that satisfies me every time. This is very freezable, so you can make a larger quantity and keep the rest to enjoy as a healthy ready meal for when you're busy. I never used to eat much onion, as it didn't agree with me, but I've been slowly reintroducing it to my diet... which is why you're now seeing more of it, too. If you're not an onion person, feel free to leave it out though.

Serves 6

NUT-FREE

large glug of olive oil

2 celery sticks, finely chopped

1 medium onion, finely chopped (optional)

salt and pepper

4 garlic cloves, finely chopped

2 red chillies, deseeded and finely chopped

400g can of chopped tomatoes

4 tablespoons tomato purée

2 red peppers, finely chopped

400g can each of butter beans, black beans
   and cannellini beans, drained and rinsed

large handful of fresh coriander

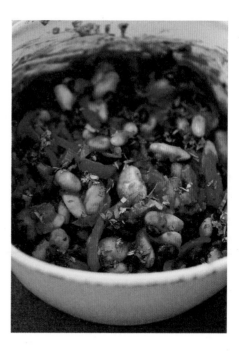

Heat the oil in a large saucepan over a medium heat. Add the celery and onion (if using) with lots of salt and pepper, then stir. Cook until the celery is turning translucent, then add the garlic and chillies and cook for a minute, stirring so that nothing catches.

Add the canned tomatoes, tomato purée, red peppers and 350ml of water and let it bubble for about 30 minutes, stirring to break down the tomatoes now and then, until the sauce is starting to reduce and the peppers are soft.

Once you're ready to eat, add the beans. They'll need about 10 minutes. When they've had that, turn the heat off and let cool slightly.

Serve in bowls with some Mango Salsa (page 143) mixed through each serving, topped with a sprinkling of coriander.

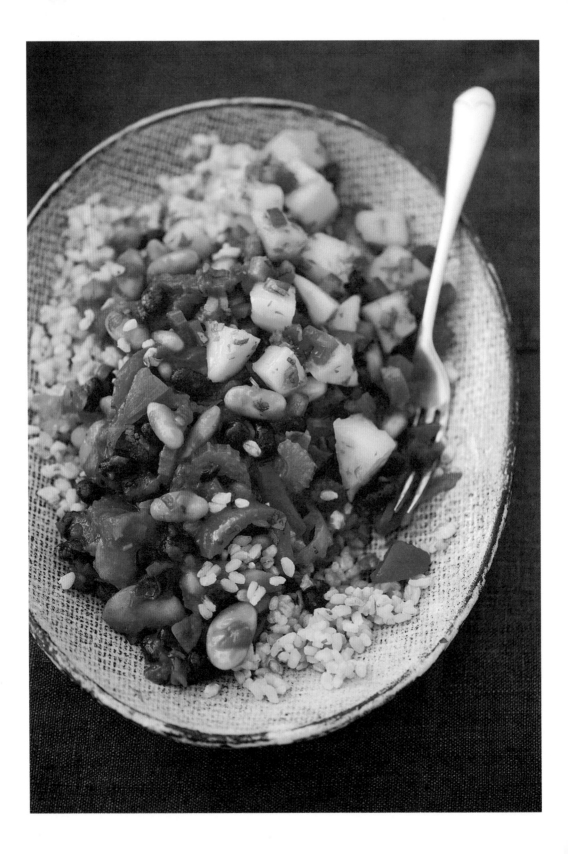

MANGO SALSA

It may sound weird to add a mango salsa to a bean stew, but trust me, it tastes incredible. It's a lovely twist to the recipe that gives a zing to each bite. It sweetens it and freshens it up, while also adding great colour, which makes the dish look much more beautiful, so your friends and family will want to devour the whole thing! You can also use this to add zip to Smoky Baked Tortilla Chips or as a summery filling for Quesadillas (pages 199 and 110). If you like onion, try a little very finely chopped sweet red onion mixed through it, too, to add a little bite.

Serves 6

NUT-FREE

3 ripe mangos

1 red pepper, deseeded

1 jalapeño or other chilli, deseeded and
    finely chopped

juice of 2 limes

1 teaspoon apple cider vinegar

3 tablespoons olive oil

salt

small handful of fresh coriander leaves,
    finely chopped

Peel the mangos, then chop into bite-sized pieces, discarding the stones. Chop the red pepper into small pieces (you want these to be smaller than the mango pieces).

Mix the mangos, pepper, jalapeño, lime juice, vinegar, olive oil and salt in a bowl. Stir well so everything is coated in oil and lime juice.

Sprinkle the coriander on top.

SUPER SPEEDY

10 minutes

CHICKPEA CHILLI IN BAKED SWEET POTATOES

This is one of my go-to easy meals, it is easy to throw together and you just need a couple of fresh ingredients to make it; everything else is a storecupboard essential, so you save money and put what you already have to good use. I promise it's still bursting with flavour though, thanks to the blend of spices, miso, garlic and chilli. I love cooking big batches of this to serve with a big pile of Spiced Roast Cauliflower on the side (page 149); it's such a warming, comforting meal and great to serve to a bunch of hungry friends. I freeze any chilli leftovers to make sure I always have some healthy instant meals on hand. If you want to eat more quickly, use quinoa instead of baked sweet potatoes, as quinoa only takes about fifteen minutes to cook.

Serves 4

NUT-FREE

FOR THE POTATOES

4 medium sweet potatoes, scrubbed well

drizzle of olive oil

sea salt flakes

FOR THE CHILLI

2 red chillies, finely chopped

2 celery sticks, finely chopped

olive oil

4 garlic cloves, crushed

1 teaspoon miso paste

2 teaspoons mustard seeds

2 teaspoons paprika

2 teaspoons ground cumin

½ teaspoon chilli powder

salt and pepper

300g cherry tomatoes, quartered

400g can of chopped tomatoes

3 tablespoons tomato purée

2 x 400g cans of chickpeas,
    drained and rinsed

2 tablespoons apple cider vinegar

200g spinach

coconut yogurt, to serve

Preheat the oven to 220°C (fan 200°C).

Place the sweet potatoes on a baking tray lined with baking parchment and pierce the skin of each on both sides, making small cuts to make sure the air can escape as they bake.

Pour a little olive oil into your hands and rub the sweet potatoes all over so they have a thin coating. Put them back on the baking tray and sprinkle sea salt flakes evenly on them on all sides.

Pop them in the oven and cook for 1 hour, until tender inside.

Meanwhile, make the chilli. Place the chillies and celery in a large frying pan over a medium-high heat with a generous glug of olive oil, adding the garlic, miso, mustard seeds, paprika, cumin, chilli, salt and pepper. Let this cook for about 5 minutes, until the celery has softened.

Add the cherry tomatoes, canned tomatoes and tomato purée, then carefully stir in the chickpeas and vinegar.

Let everything cook for about 30 minutes. When you're ready to eat, stir though the spinach to wilt. Check the seasoning again, then serve the chilli with the baked sweet potatoes and a dollop of coconut yogurt.

MIX IT UP

Try baked sweet potatoes filled with Maple & Rosemary Butter Beans (page 51).

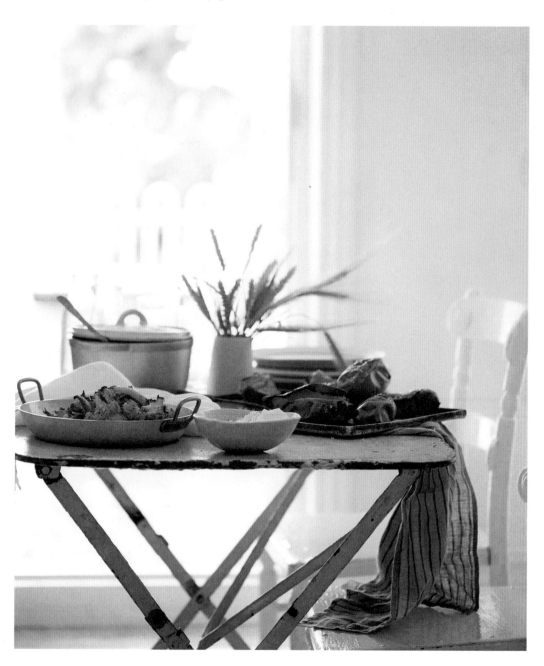

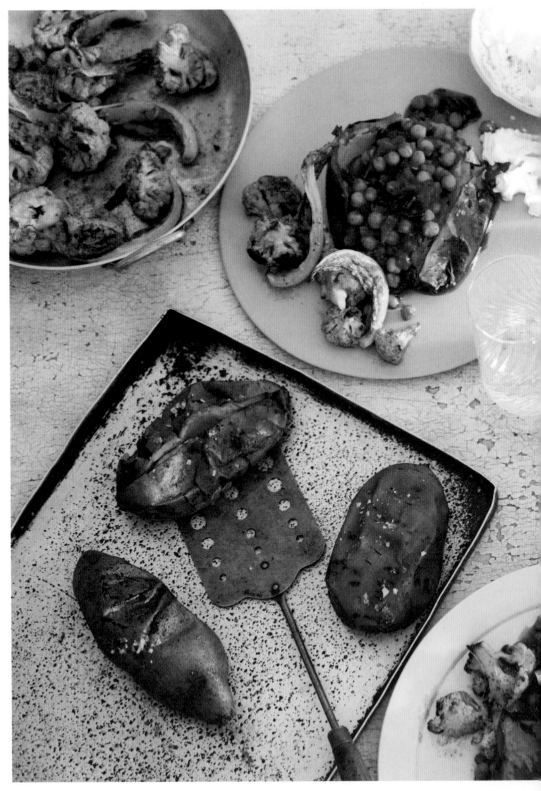

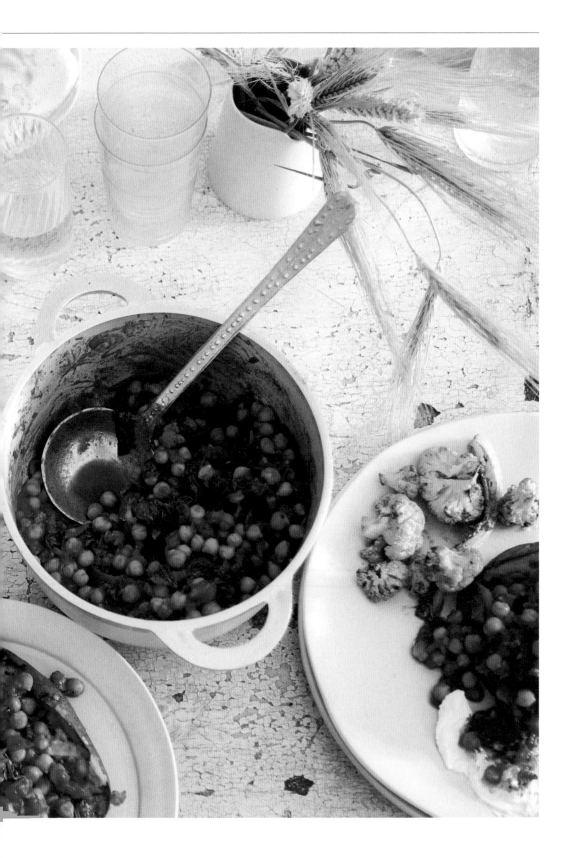

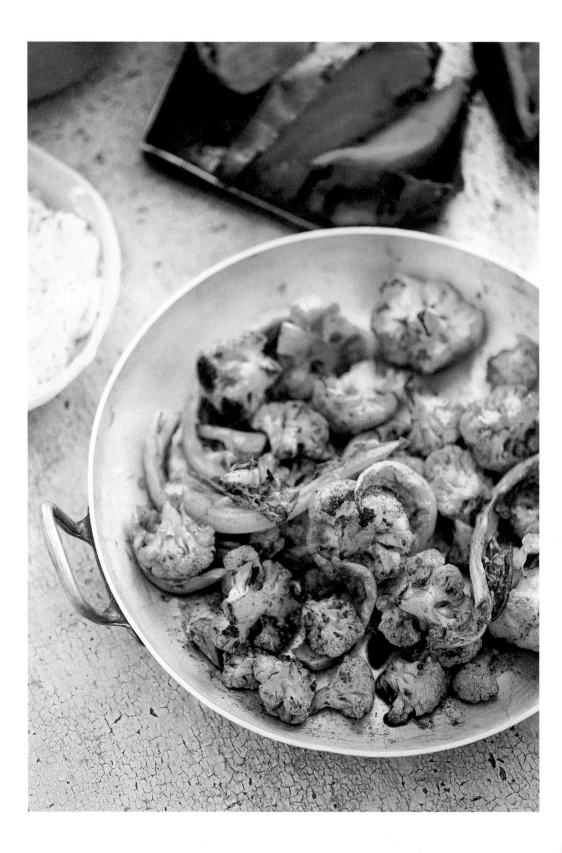

SPICED ROAST CAULIFLOWER

Caulifower is one of the best vegetables because it's so versatile. It's particularly delicious when it's roasted with lots of warming spices until it turns golden brown and slightly crispy; like this, it's almost unbeatable. The spices do wonders here to make sure that every bite is bursting with flavour, plus they really complement the spices used in the Chickpea Chilli (page 144), which is why the dishes go so well together.

Serves 4 as a side dish

NUT-FREE

3 tablespoons olive oil
1 teaspoon ground turmeric
½ teaspoon cayenne pepper
½ teaspoon ground cumin
salt and lots of pepper
1 cauliflower, broken into florets

Preheat the oven to 220°C (fan 200°C).

In a large bowl, combine the oil and the spices, mix with a whisk, then toss in the cauliflower florets. Use spoons to toss if you'd prefer not to get turmeric all over your fingers! (It can stain them yellow.) The cauliflower florets should be coated all over in the spiced oil.

Pour the spicy cauliflower out on to a baking sheet and roast for 35–40 minutes until the pieces are golden brown.

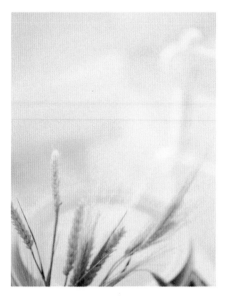

MY FAVOURITE CURRIED VEGGIES

The best meal for a cosy night snuggled on the sofa. Each mouthful is bursting with flavour, as the carrots, peppers, cauliflower, peas and spinach are cooked in an amazing blend of coconut milk and spices. I love serving this in a big bowl with a bed of hot brown rice under the curry and a good dollop of my Lime & Chilli Pickle on the side (page 153). This tastes even better the next day, if you don't finish it all in one sitting.

Serves 3–4 generously

NUT-FREE

1 medium cauliflower, broken into similar-sized florets

4 tablespoons olive oil

salt and pepper

4 carrots, peeled and sliced into 2.5cm chunks on the diagonal

2 red peppers, deseeded and chopped into 2.5cm chunks

2 tablespoons cumin seeds

5 garlic cloves, finely grated

5cm root ginger, finely grated

½ teaspoon ground turmeric

3 teaspoons ground coriander

2 teaspoons ground cumin

1 tablespoon curry powder

5 cloves

3 tablespoons tomato purée

400g can of chopped tomatoes

400ml can of coconut milk

2 green finger chillies

juice of ½ lemon, or to taste

200g fresh baby spinach

100g frozen peas

large handful of fresh coriander leaves, chopped

Preheat the oven to 210°C (fan 190°C). Take 2 baking sheets or trays. Place the cauliflower on the first tray, drizzle with 1 tablespoon of oil, season with salt and pepper and give them a mix to evenly coat. Place the carrots and peppers on the second tray, drizzle with 1 tablespoon of oil, salt and pepper and the cumin seeds, mix it all with your hands, then roast both trays for 45 minutes. Check every 10 minutes or so, and give them a shake; you want the carrots and pepper to shrivel and sweeten, and the cauliflower to blacken a little and take on a gorgeous roasted flavour.

Meanwhile, in a high-sided pot, gently heat the remaining 2 tablespoons of olive oil, then add the garlic and ginger with a pinch of salt and stir so it cooks a little but doesn't colour. Once they give off a lovely scent, add the rest of the dry spices and stir, still making sure not to burn anything. Add the tomato purée and stir again, then the canned tomatoes and coconut milk. Bring to the boil and let it simmer gently. Add the green chillies. If you're like me and enjoy spicy food, slice them open and leave the seeds in; however, for a milder curry, throw them in whole. The longer you leave it simmering, the more delicious it will taste, but I cook it for at least 30 minutes.

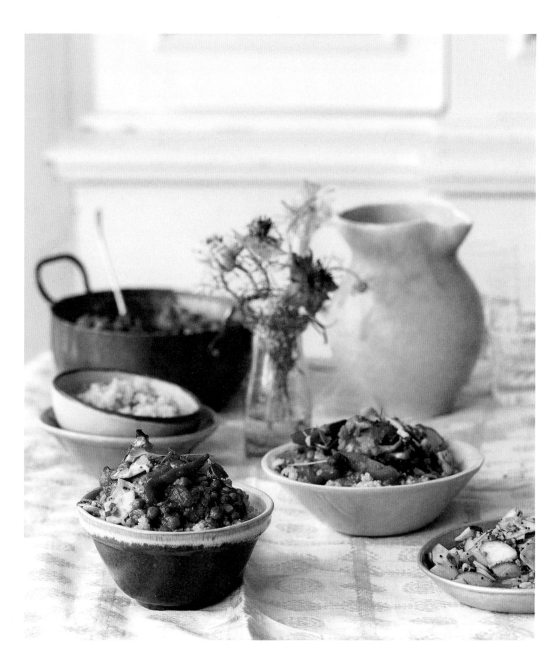

When there are just 5 minutes before you want to eat, taste the curry and add lemon juice to heighten the flavours. Stir in the spinach and peas, they should take about 2 minutes to wilt and defrost. Finally, stir in the roasted vegetables, being careful not to break the cauliflower florets apart too much.

Serve with brown rice or quinoa, sprinkling with lots of fresh coriander before eating.

CLEVER COOKING
I don't bother to peel ginger, just grate it straight into the pan.

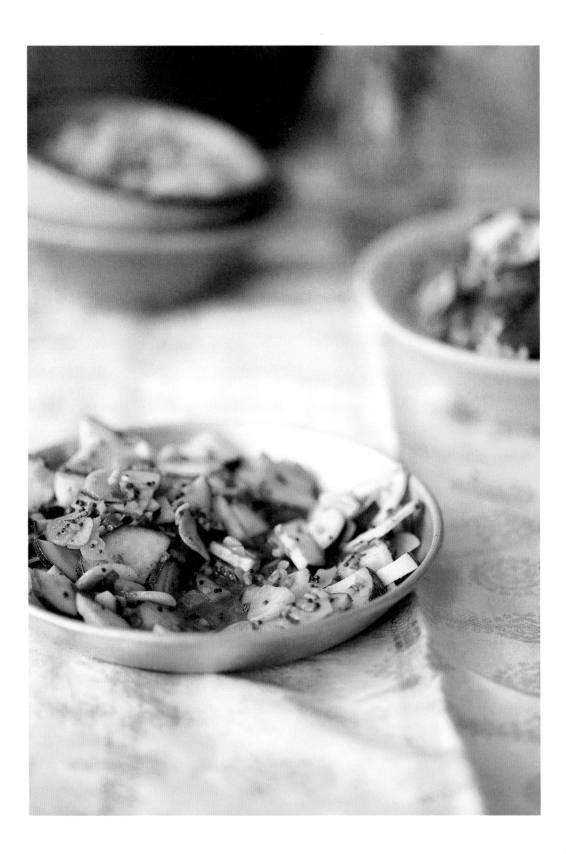

LIME & CHILLI PICKLE

This is a great addition to My Favourite Curried Veggies (page 150); it really brings out so much of the flavour and heightens all the amazing essences of the meal. The mix of mustard and fenugreek seeds with the other spices is just incredible, especially with the zesty lime and apple cider vinegar. I'm sure you'll love the taste of this. You can add a dollop to any meal, not only a curry, to add an extra punch to a simple dish.

Makes enough for 3–4

NUT-FREE

1 teaspoon mustard seeds

½ teaspoon fenugreek seeds

8 garlic cloves

knob of root ginger

1–2 red chillies (depending on how spicy you like it)

2 tablespoons toasted sesame oil

1 teaspoon ground turmeric

1 teaspoon chilli powder

1 teaspoon ground coriander

juice of 3 limes

2 tablespoons apple cider vinegar

1 courgette

Place a frying pan over a medium heat and dry fry the mustard seeds and fenugreek seeds for about 2 minutes, or until fragrant, then set aside in a bowl.

Peel and finely slice the garlic cloves, peel and finely chop the ginger and chop the chillies, then add them all to the frying pan with the sesame oil. Cook, stirring continuously, for about 5 minutes, until the garlic and ginger are cooked through and just starting to brown.

Add the mustard seeds, fenugreek seeds, ground spices, lime juice and vinegar and cook for another minute

Cut the courgette into quarters lengthways, then finely slice. Add this to the frying pan (you can add 1 tablespoon of water if things are starting to stick), and cook for a further 6–8 minutes, or until cooked through.

Remove from the heat and allow to cool before serving.

CLEVER COOKING

If by any chance you have made the pickle too spicy, then add a cooling dollop of coconut yogurt, it tastes delicious and is far more effective than water for removing chilli burn.

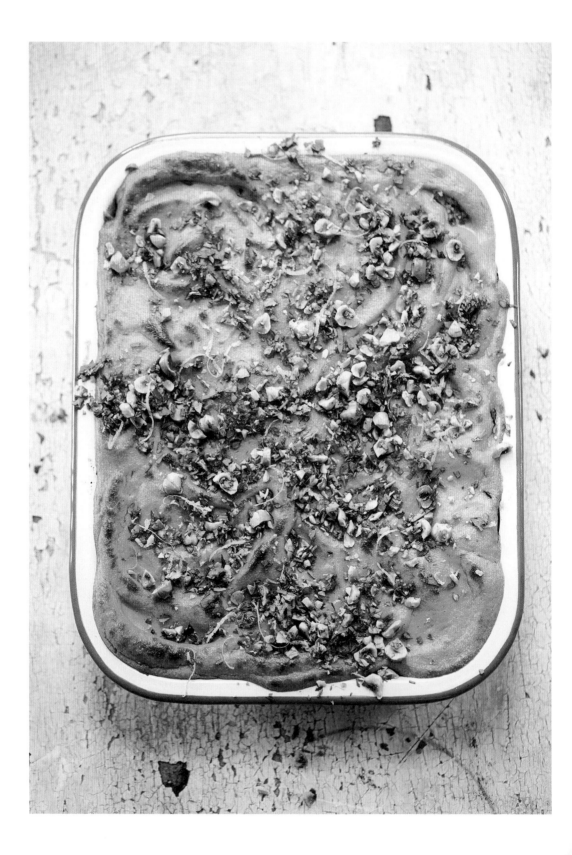

TOMATO & AUBERGINE BAKE

This is one of my favourite recipes in the book, it's really very special and I'd recommend you all trying it as soon as you can! The 'cheesy' layer, which was inspired by the amazing Serena in my office, is the best part. It makes each bite so creamy and rich, warming and comforting... perfect for a cold evening with friends. I find this filling enough on its own, so I normally just make a side of Spinach with Mustard Seeds (page 156) to sit alongside it, but it's great with some hot quinoa, too.

Serves 6–8

2 large aubergines

lots of salt and pepper

2 courgettes

3 tablespoons olive oil, plus more to brush

1 fennel bulb, finely chopped

3 red peppers, deseeded, roughly chopped

6 garlic cloves, crushed

4 teaspoons smoked paprika

3 x 400g cans of chopped tomatoes

2 tablespoons tomato puree

280g jar of sun-dried tomatoes in oil (170g
    drained weight), drained and chopped

a few sprigs of thyme

1 teaspoon chilli flakes

100g hazelnuts

finely grated zest of 1 unwaxed lemon

25g flat leaf parsley, leaves picked and
    finely chopped

FOR THE CHEESY SAUCE

200g butternut squash (about one-third
    of a squash)

150g cashew nuts, soaked in water for at
    least 4 hours, then drained

2 tablespoons nutritional yeast

3 teaspoons tamari

½ teaspoon cayenne pepper (optional)

juice of 1 lemon

Preheat the oven to 180°C (fan 160°C).

Slice the aubergines lengthways into slices roughly 5mm thick, place on 2 baking trays in a single layer, sprinkle liberally with salt and set aside to let water draw out. Slice the courgettes lengthways into 5mm slices too.

Place a griddle pan over a high heat. Brush it with olive oil and start griddling the courgette slices. Lay them on gently and leave them until you can see the griddle lines coming through the top side. Set aside. Keep going until all the courgettes are done.

Get started on your tomato sauce. Heat about 3 tablespoons of olive oil in a large non-stick frying pan and add the chopped fennel with salt and pepper. Sauté for about 3 minutes over a medium heat before adding the peppers and garlic, and sauté for another 3 minutes before adding the paprika, stirring to coat. Now tip in the canned tomatoes, tomato purée, sun-dried tomatoes, thyme and chilli flakes. Let this simmer and reduce for at least 20 minutes.

Meanwhile you can get on with the aubergines. Using kitchen paper, brush off the salt and water from the aubergine slices, and start griddling on the hot griddle (make   >>

sure you have your extractor fan on! It gets smoky but the flavour makes it worthwhile). Griddle for about 1 minute each side, and set aside. Once the aubergines are all done, the sauce should have reduced by one-third, look glossy and coat the back of a spoon nicely. If this is so, you can start assembling the bake. Check the sauce for seasoning and add more salt and pepper if needed.

Place the hazelnuts on a shallow roasting tray and roast for 7–10 minutes, so that they turn golden. Set aside to cool

Take a lasagne dish and put a layer of aubergine on the bottom, followed by a layer of tomato sauce, then a layer of courgettes and keep layering until everything is used up, finishing with a layer of the tomato sauce.

Cover with foil and place in the middle shelf of the oven for 30 minutes.

Now make your cheesy sauce by peeling, roughly chopping and steaming the squash for 15 minutes. Then simply blend all the ingredients in a high-speed blender until totally smooth, seasoning very well.

Remove the foil from the bake, pour over the sauce and cook for another 10 minutes.

Meanwhile, chop the hazelnuts and mix in a bowl with the lemon zest and parsley.

Remove the bake from the oven, sprinkle half of the herby nut mixture over the top and take to the table to serve. Put the rest of the hazelnut mixture in a bowl on the table so people can add extra to their plate should they want it.

CLEVER COOK
Keep lemons after you have zested them to slice and use in drinks, such as in a big jug of water for the table.

SPINACH WITH MUSTARD SEEDS

I love serving a big bowl of this hot, wilted spinach as a side in the winter. Sautéing the spinach with mustard seeds, garlic, lemon and ginger gives it so much flavour, but the quantities of each ingredient aren't huge so the taste isn't overpowering, allowing the dish to always complement your main. I think it's the perfect addition to my favourite Tomato & Aubergine Bake (page 155), plus it adds another portion of veg to the meal, which means you can get the goodness from six different veggies!

Serves 6

NUT-FREE

600g 'adult' (not baby leaf) spinach

3 tablespoons olive oil

3 teaspoons mustard seeds

3 garlic cloves, crushed

6cm root ginger, finely grated

juice of 1½ lemons

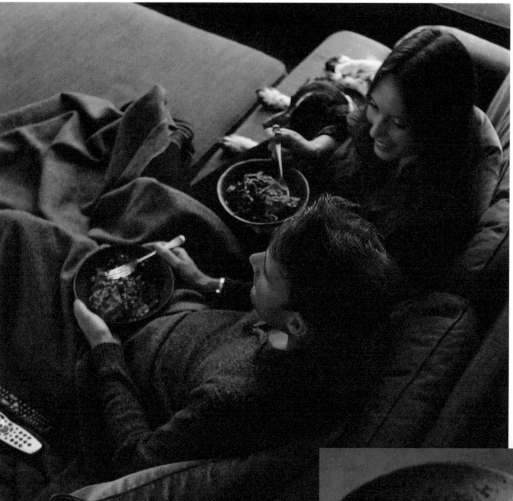

First rinse the spinach, then roughly chop it.

Heat the oil in a large frying pan. Once it's hot, add the mustard seeds and cook them until they start to pop, then add the garlic and ginger and stir, making sure the garlic doesn't colour, for about 1 minute.

Throw in the spinach and squeeze in the lemon juice, cook until the spinach is wilted, then enjoy straight away.

PAN TO PLATE
10 minutes

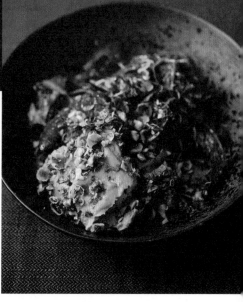

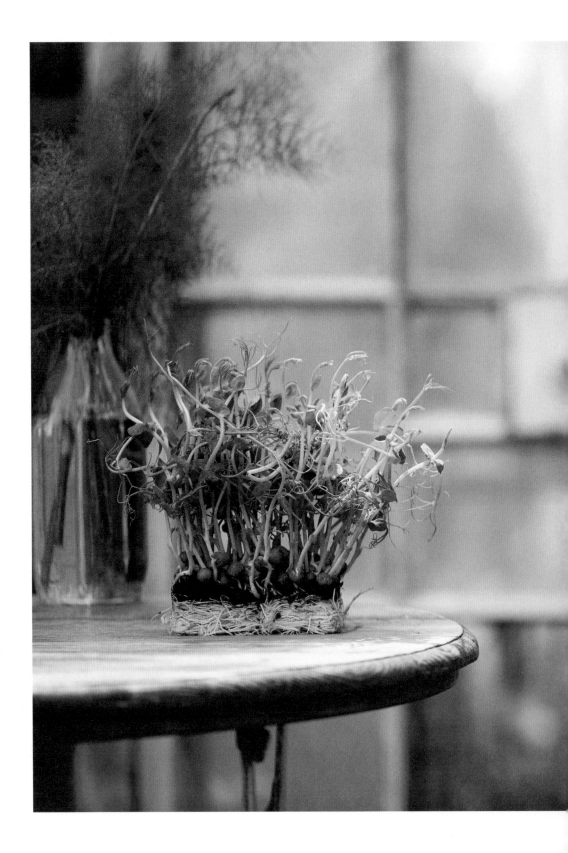

SIDES

VIBRANT BOWLS OF GOODNESS TO ADD TO ANY MEAL

WHOLE ROASTED CUMIN & DATE CARROTS

I had the most amazing whole roasted carrots with dates in a restaurant in LA a few years ago, and I loved them so much that I had to recreate them the next day and have made them many times ever since. I add a little maple syrup to the carrots as they roast to enhance their sweetness, plus some paprika and cumin to intensify the flavours. These taste amazing with everything, but they're particularly good alongside the Miso & Sesame Glazed Aubergines (page 173). If you can get carrots in different colours, they look great.

Serves 4 as a side dish

NUT-FREE

16 small carrots (about 650g), I use carrots with the tops still on because they look nice, peeled or well scrubbed

olive oil

1 tablespoon maple syrup

1 teaspoon ground cumin

1 teaspoon cumin seeds

1 teaspoon paprika

salt

4 medjool dates, pitted and roughly chopped

Preheat the oven to 220°C (fan 200°C).

Place the carrots on a baking tray, drizzle with a generous amount of olive oil, the maple syrup, both types of cumin, the paprika and salt. Toss the carrots in the mix, to make sure they're evenly coated.

Roast for about 30 minutes, giving the carrots a shake halfway through.

Take the tray out of the oven, add the dates and mix gently, then return to the oven for a final 10 minutes, after which the carrots should be golden, sweet and delicious... and a tad wrinkly.

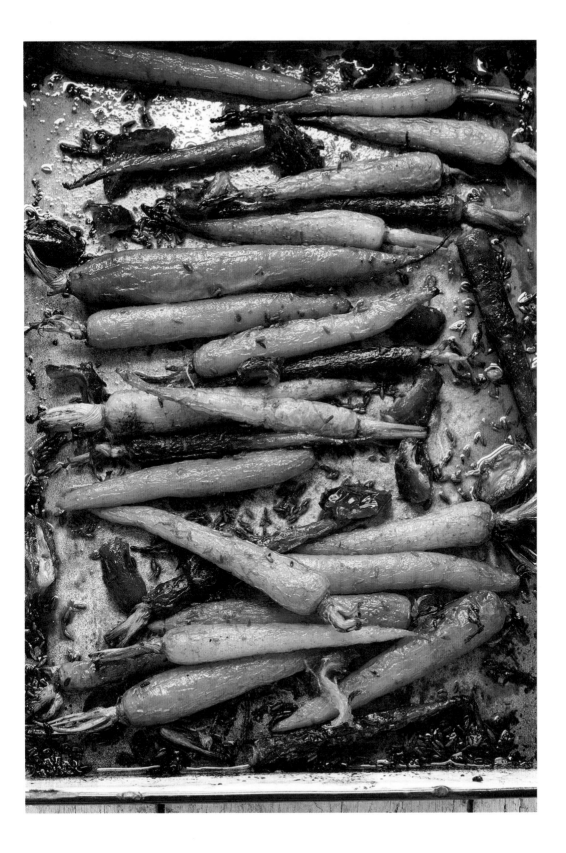

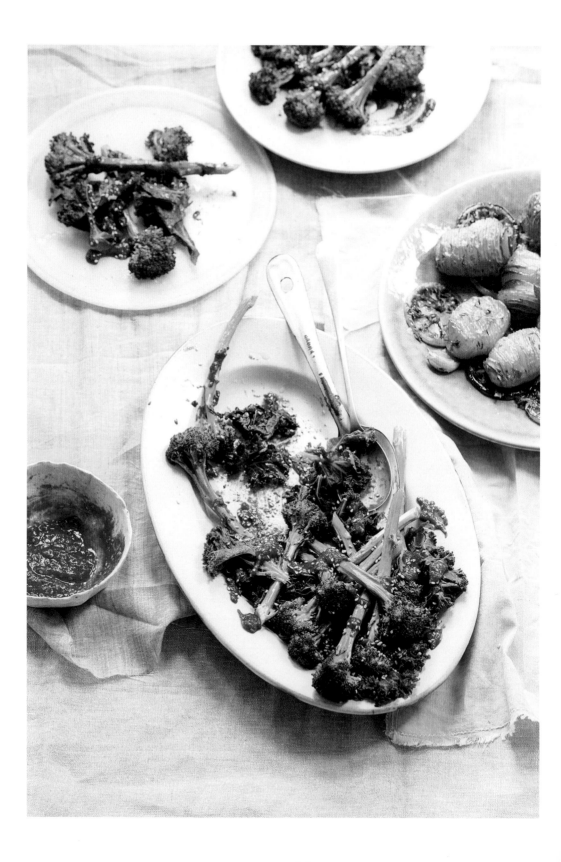

HARISSA & SESAME GREENS

This is my absolute best way to eat greens; the mix of sesame and harissa just makes them so delicious. Each bite is bursting with flavour, and the subtle spiciness does wonders for making something so simple taste really special. I eat these with so many dishes, from simple quinoa bowls to Spiced Potato Cakes with Garlicky Tomato Sauce or Herbed Nut Roast (pages 60 and 123). They also make a fantastic duo of sides with Lemony Hasselback Potatoes (page 164).

Serves 4 as a side dish

NUT-FREE

24 spears of Tenderstem broccoli
 (about 6 per person)
2 tablespoons olive oil, plus more
 to roast the broccoli
150g torn-up kale, coarse ribs removed
3 tablespoons harissa
2 teaspoons sesame seeds,
 plus more to serve
juice of ½ lemon
salt

Preheat the oven to 200°C (fan 180°C).

Place the broccoli on a baking tray and coat with a little olive oil. Toss the stems so they are lightly coated in oil. Roast for 10–15 minutes, until it is cooked and slightly charred.

Meanwhile, steam the kale. It should take about 5 minutes. Drain well.

Mix the harissa in a bowl with the sesame seeds, lemon juice, the 2 tablespoons of olive oil and salt.

Once the veg is cooked, place the kale on a plate and scatter the broccoli on top with a little more salt. Finally drizzle the harissa mix on everything and sprinkle with a few more sesame seeds to serve.

LEMONY HASSELBACK POTATOES

I made this recipe for Christmas last year and it was such a hit that I wanted to share it with you all. It's a great recipe for two reasons: firstly – obviously – they taste great as the potatoes are infused with garlic, lemon and thyme as they cook, soaking up all the flavours; but secondly they look amazing with their perfectly cut, crispy golden skin, so they'll instantly impress all your guests. The good news for you is that they're actually really easy to make, as long as you have a sharp knife and a steady hand! It's simple to double (or even triple) the recipe, as we did for this photograph.

Serves 4–6 as a side dish

NUT-FREE

8 medium roasting potatoes, scrubbed well, skins left on
1 lemon
8 garlic cloves, unpeeled and squashed (bash with a rolling pin!)
leaves from 4 sprigs of fresh thyme, plus more to serve
plenty of good olive oil
sea salt flakes and pepper

Preheat the oven to 220°C (fan 200°C).

On a chopping board, firmly hold a potato and, with a sharp knife, make cuts two-thirds of the way through it, each 1–2mm apart, depending on your patience! When you're doing this, concentrate, because you want to make sure your potato isn't cut the whole way through to the board otherwise it won't hold together. Use this time as a sort of meditation! Do this for all the spuds and then place them on a baking tray, sliced sides up.

Cut the lemon in half, then squeeze its juice over the potatoes. Now reshape the lemon to its original form as far as possible, slice it into rings and place into the baking tray. Throw in the garlic and thyme, drizzle with loads of olive oil, getting as much as you can into the cuts you've made in your spuds, sprinkle very liberally with salt flakes and pepper and roll everything around so that the potatoes are all nicely coated. Make sure they're all sitting sliced sides up again and put them in the oven.

After about 25 minutes, take out the lemon slices and garlic and set aside; you can eat the garlic with the potatoes later and the lemons make the dish look beautiful when presented, but if you leave them in the oven for the whole time they will burn to a cinder.

Spoon the juices at the bottom of the tray back over the potatoes and return them to the oven for another 60–65 minutes, until crispy on top and cooked through.

Sprinkle with fresh thyme and return the lemon slices and garlic, if you like, to serve.

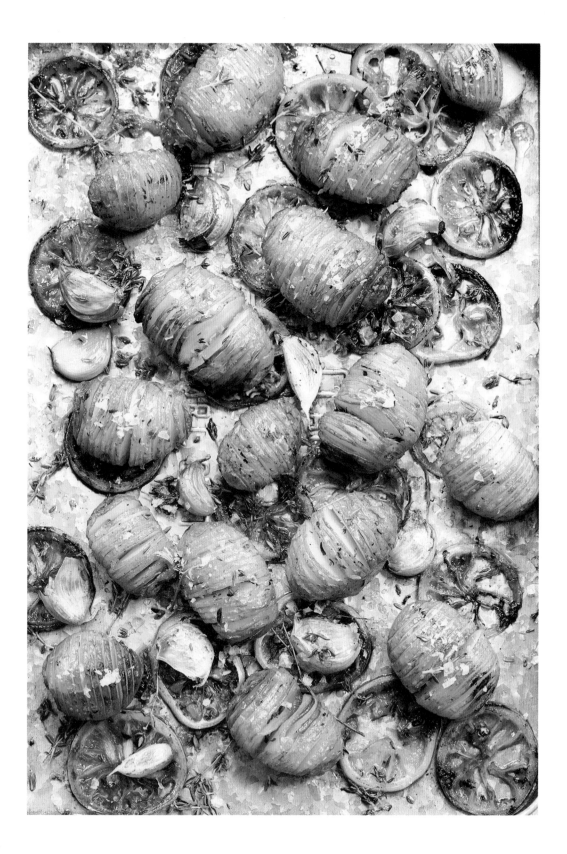

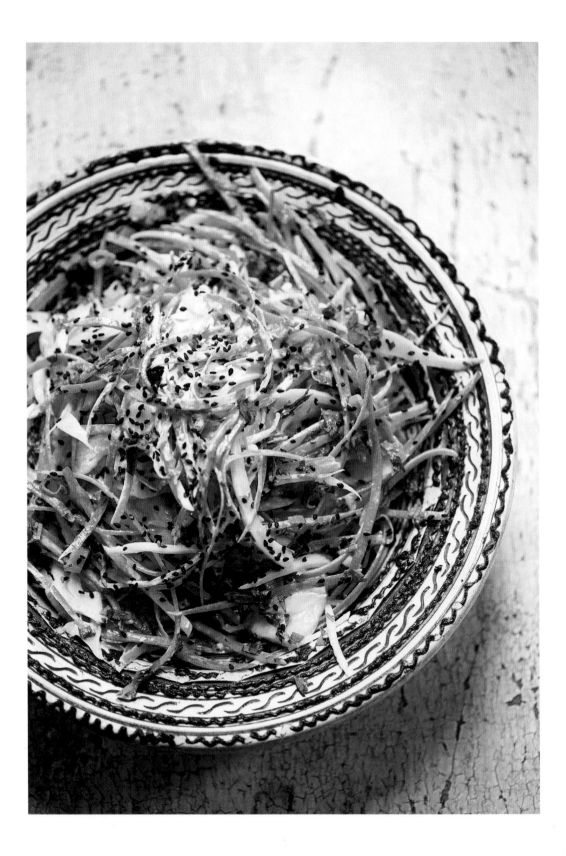

CARROT & FENNEL SLAW

This is probably the simplest, lightest recipe in this whole chapter. It's lovely and delicate, with only a handful of flavours, so that it can sit really well alongside rich dishes. I love having a side like this that I can throw together in a few minutes, to add more colour and texture to the table, but without distracting from the centrepieces of a meal.

Serves 4 as a side dish

NUT-FREE

2 tablespoons olive oil

1 tablespoon toasted sesame oil

4 tablespoons coconut yogurt

2 tablespoons apple cider vinegar

juice of ½ lemon

salt and pepper

1 small fennel bulb

2 medium carrots, peeled

4 spring onions

2 tablespoons black sesame seeds

handful of chopped fresh coriander

Place the olive oil, sesame oil, yogurt, vinegar and lemon juice in a mixing bowl and whisk vigorously to make an emulsion, then season with salt and pepper.

Trim the base of the fennel bulb and, using a mandolin, slice it as thin as possible. (If you don't have a mandolin, just slice it very thinly with a knife.) Place the sliced fennel into the bowl with the dressing.

Next, slice the carrots on the mandolin, or use a shredder, so they resemble ribbons or shreds; if you don't have a mandolin, use a vegetable peeler to make ribbons. You want the carrot to retain a bit of crunch, so it's better to take the time to do this, rather than just grating it. Place in the bowl with the fennel and dressing and mix with your hands so everything is coated nicely.

Finely chop the spring onions and mix them into the slaw.

Sprinkle with the sesame seeds and chopped coriander and serve.

SUPER SPEEDY

10 minutes

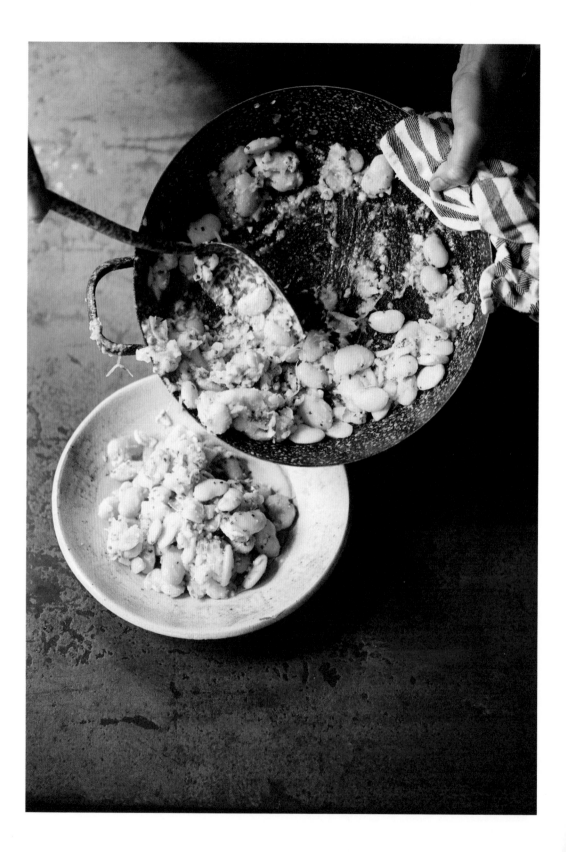

ZESTY BUTTER BEANS

This is a wonderfully simple, subtle side dish. The beans have a deliciously delicate flavour with subtle hints of rosemary, lemon and cayenne. None of the flavours are overpowering, so they'll complement your main dish perfectly, and are especially good with my Spiced Potato Cakes with Garlicky Tomato Sauce, or Sesame, Coriander & Roasted Fennel Rice Bowl, or with a big pile of Harissa & Sesame Greens and some Smoky Babaganoush on the side (pages 60, 104, 163 and 203).

Serves 4

NUT-FREE

olive oil

6 garlic cloves, crushed

6 sprigs of rosemary, leaves stripped
and roughly chopped

2 x 400g cans of butter beans, drained
and rinsed

finely grated zest of 1 unwaxed lemon,
plus the juice of 1½ lemons

½ teaspoon cayenne pepper

salt and pepper

Add a big glug of olive oil to a saucepan, place over a medium heat and heat it up, then add the garlic and rosemary. Let this cook for 3–5 minutes, until it's bubbling away.

Add the beans, lemon zest and juice and cayenne pepper and cook for 5–10 minutes, until the beans are soft. As you're stirring the beans, crush them slightly so you end up with a part-whole-bean-part-creamy-mash mix. Season to taste.

Drizzle with another glug of olive oil, to stop them becoming dry, then serve.

SUPER SPEEDY
10 minutes

BLACKENED CAULIFLOWER
WITH SPRING ONION PESTO

Pesto instantly adds colour and flavour to anything, plus it's always so quick and easy to whizz together. As I make it so much, I love to try different variations, and this spring onion version is a real winner. I can't tell you how good it tastes with the blackened cauliflower. I like to make extra pesto, so that I can keep a bowl in the fridge for a few days ready to stir though pasta or beans for a quick go-to meal.

Serves 4 as a side dish

NUT-FREE

FOR THE CAULIFLOWER

1 cauliflower, broken into florets

olive oil

salt and pepper

FOR THE PESTO

bunch of spring onions, green tops only

50g pine nuts

10g fresh basil leaves

3 tablespoons nutritional yeast

1 garlic clove, crushed

juice of ½ lemon

100ml olive oil

Preheat the oven to 180°C (fan 160°C).

Place the cauliflower florets on a baking tray, drizzle with a little olive oil, season with salt and pepper, and pop them into the oven. Set a timer for 40 minutes, but check them every 10 minutes or so and give them a shake every now and again. You want them to blacken and char slightly on all sides.

Meanwhile, make the pesto. Boil the kettle while you chop the spring onion tops and place them in a colander. Pour boiling water over the spring onion tops so that they wilt.

Put the pine nuts, basil, nutritional yeast, garlic, lemon juice and wilted spring onion tops into a food processor and blend. Once it has become a paste, slowly pour in the oil while the processor is still running. Season with salt and pepper to taste.

Once the cauliflower is cooked, serve on a platter or in a shallow dish and dollop and drizzle the spring onion pesto on top (or serve it in a bowl on the side, if you prefer). Enjoy!

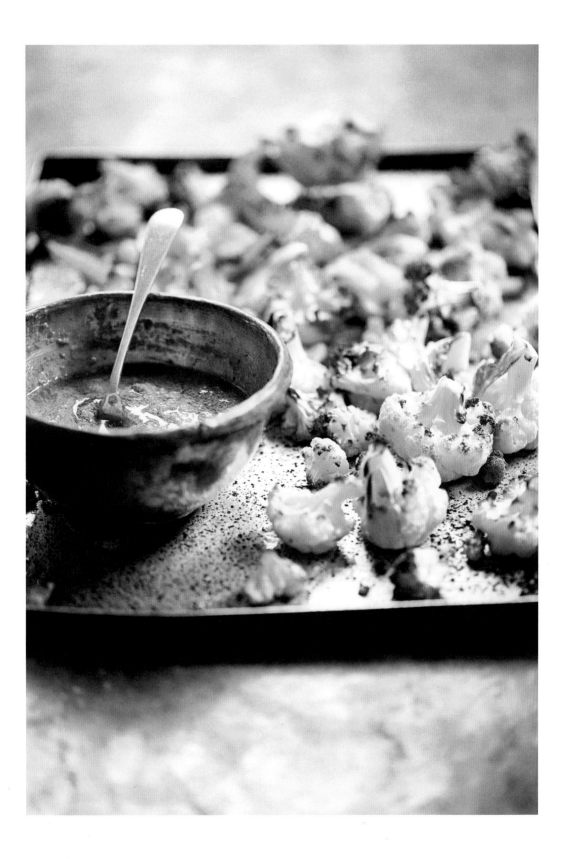

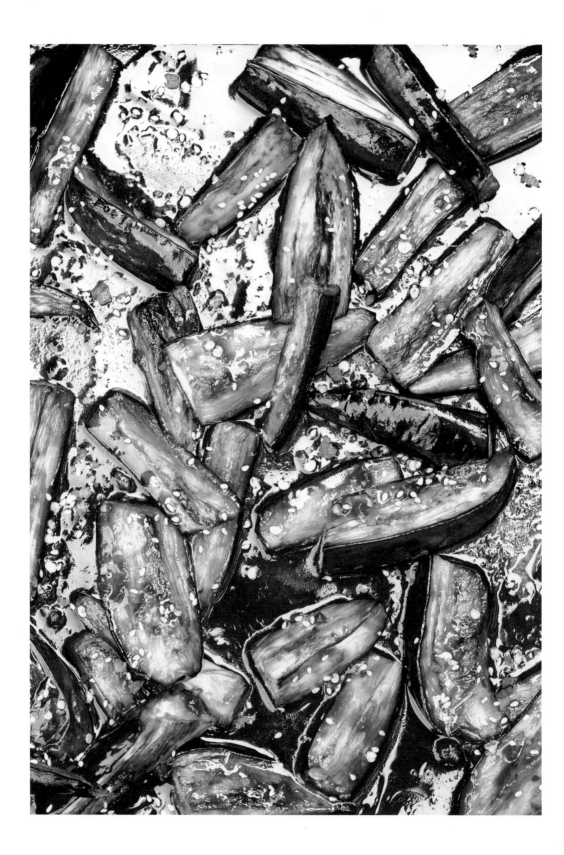

MISO & SESAME GLAZED AUBERGINES

*These aubergine wedges are one of the most popular recipes I've created for this book.
I've made them for so many friends and everyone goes crazy for them and asks for them
again and again. They're so insanely delicious. The mix of sesame, tamari, miso, maple
and lemon juice creates such rich flavours that really make each bite sing! I always make
extra as everyone seems to want seconds, but also because they taste great cold, so I throw
any leftovers into my lunch box the next day.*

Serves 4 as a side dish

NUT-FREE

FOR THE AUBERGINES

3 medium aubergines, stalks removed,
    cut into small wedges lengthways

1 tablespoon olive oil

salt

sesame seeds, to serve

chilli flakes, to serve

FOR THE GLAZE

3 tablespoons toasted sesame oil

1½ tablespoons tamari

2 teaspoons brown rice miso

1 tablespoon maple syrup

juice of 1 lemon

1 teaspoon apple cider vinegar

Preheat the oven to 200°C (fan 180°C).

Place the aubergine wedges on a baking
tray, drizzle with the olive oil and sprinkle with
a little salt. Bake for 15–20 minutes, until soft
but not completely cooked.

Meanwhile, whisk the glaze ingredients
together in a bowl.

Once the wedges are soft, pour the glaze
over them (while they're still on the baking
tray) and mix well. Return them to the oven
to cook for another 10 minutes, then turn
them over and cook for a final 5 minutes until
they're tender and delicious and completely
coated in the glaze.

Take out of the oven and sprinkle with
sesame seeds and chilli flakes to serve.

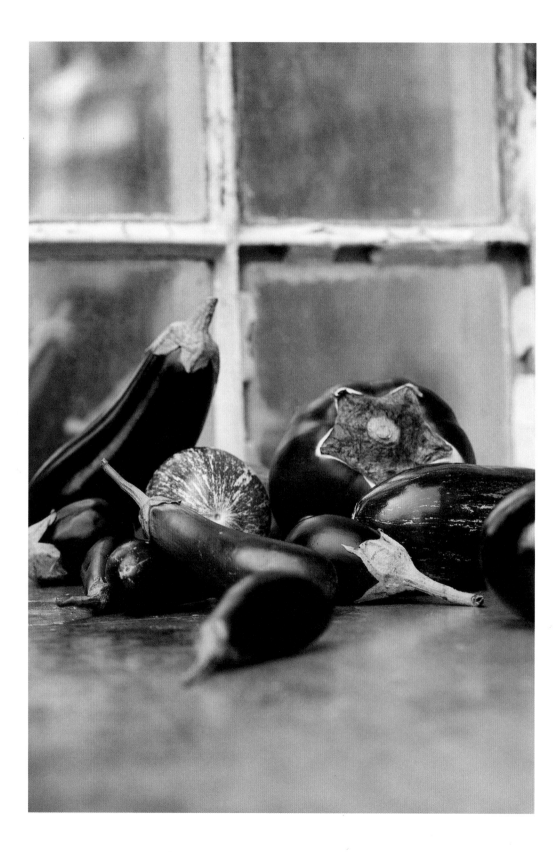

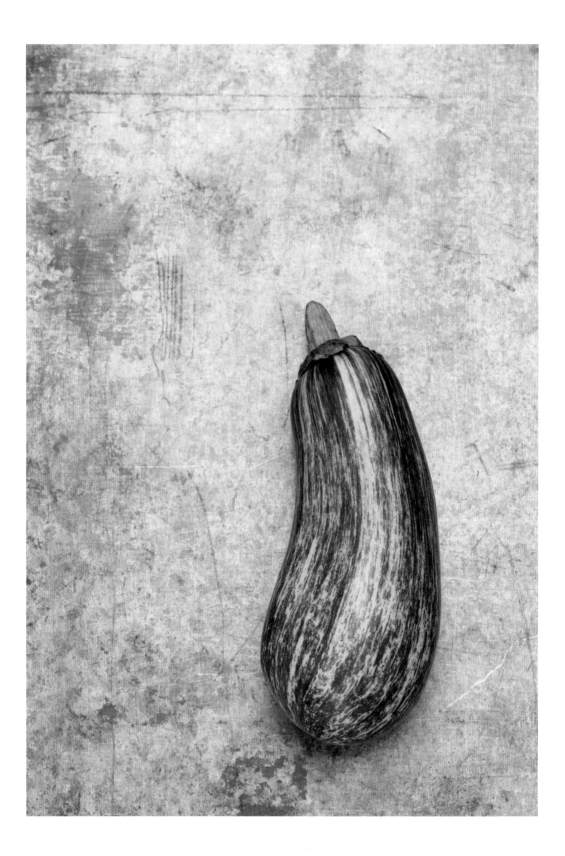

WARM MOROCCAN CAULIFLOWER 'RICE' SALAD

This is a firm favourite in the Deliciously Ella office. It's inspired by the lovely Jess, in my office, and I hope you love it as much as we do. I've always been a bit sceptical about cauliflower rice, but it's growing on me and – used in this way – I think it's great. The rice is sautéed in a warming mix of spices, then tossed with roasted cashews, apricots, raisins and chickpeas, which together create something quite outstanding. I love it with Whole Roasted Cumin & Date Carrots (page 160).

Serves 4–6 as a side dish

FOR THE SALAD

100g cashews

1 large cauliflower (about 1kg)

2 tablespoons olive oil

400g can of chickpeas, drained and rinsed

2 teaspoons ground turmeric

2 teaspoons ground cumin

2 teaspoons cumin seeds

2 teaspoons ground coriander

½ teaspoon ground cinnamon

½ teaspoon chilli powder

1 teaspoon paprika

salt and pepper

75g raisins

200g dried apricots (preferably
    unsulphured), roughly chopped

4 spring onions, finely chopped

50g fresh mint, leaves picked and chopped

50g fresh flat leaf parsley, leaves picked
    and chopped

FOR THE DRESSING

2 tablespoons tahini

1½ tablespoons olive oil

juice of ½ lemon

juice of ½ orange

Preheat the oven to 200°C (fan 180°C). Place the cashews on a baking tray and roast for 5–10 minutes until they turn golden brown. Remove from the oven and leave to cool.

Cut the cauliflower florets from the stem and chop into 2.5–5cm pieces. This makes 'ricing' them much easier. Place in a food processor. Blitz until they start to resemble rice; this should take about 30 seconds.

Heat the olive oil in a large frying pan. Add the cauliflower and chickpeas, spices, salt and pepper. Give it a good mix, then add the raisins, apricots and cashews. Mix in the pan for about 5 minutes until it's all warmed up. Remove the pan from the heat.

Meanwhile, whisk all the dressing ingredients in a bowl. Check the seasoning of the cauliflower, then mix in the spring onions and herbs. Drizzle with the dressing and enjoy!

MIX IT UP

I sometimes like this with a dollop of coconut yogurt and a pinch of the Moroccan spice blend *ras el hanout* on top.

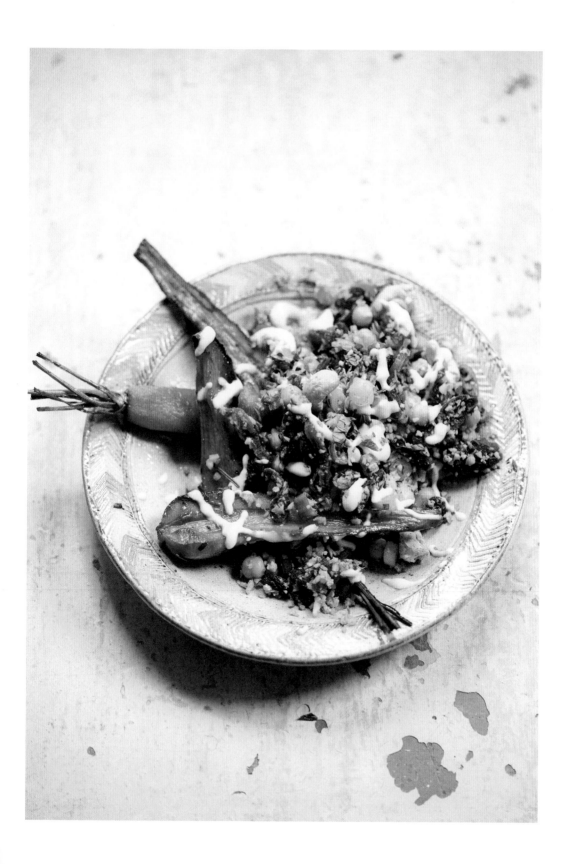

MINTY PEA PURÉE

This has been a family favourite for ages, I make it all the time when I'm at my Mum's. It's another unassuming dish that doesn't require much time or effort, but the flavours are amazing. It is one of the quick fixes I reach for when I'm short on time and want to speedily make something delicious for us at home. I'll often just heat up some quinoa, roast some broccoli, sauté some beans (such as my Zesty Butter Beans, page 169), then throw it all together for a speedy supper.

Serves 4–6 as a side dish

NUT-FREE

500g frozen peas
6 tablespoons olive oil
juice of 1½ limes, or to taste (I often
   use a little more)
small handful of fresh mint leaves
   (about 10g), roughly chopped
salt and pepper

Place the peas in a pan of cold water. Put the lid on the pan and bring it to the boil, then simmer for 2 minutes. Drain, then place in a food processor with all the other ingredients.

Whizz everything together until it's fully blended, then serve. This tastes great either served warm, or left to cool.

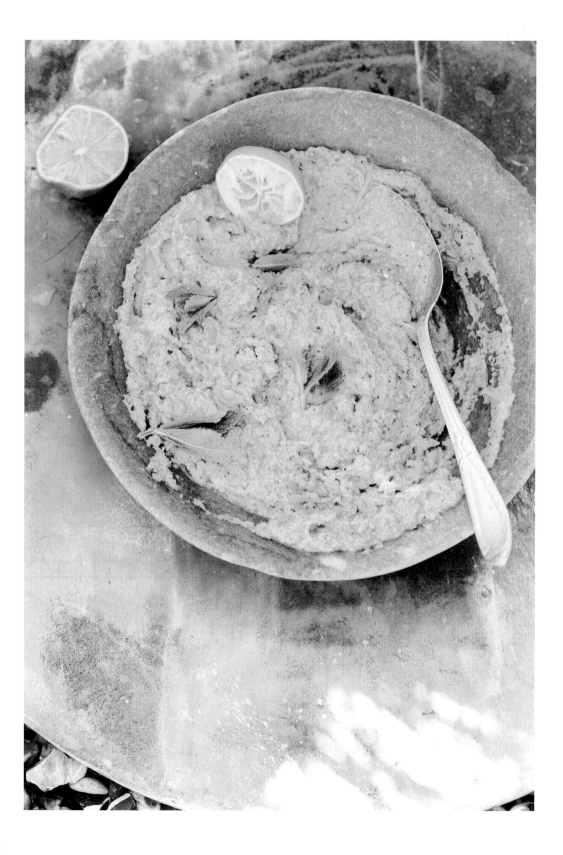

SMASHED TURMERIC & MUSTARD SEED POTATOES

This is almost my favourite dish in the chapter. Everything about these potatoes is incredibly warming and comforting; they always make me feel so grounded and happy. They are boiled and then smashed with spices, lemon juice, olive oil and lots of salt and pepper. I know lots of people stay away from potatoes, but you have to try these, they'll totally convert you into fans of the humble little spud.

Serves 4 as a side dish

NUT-FREE

1kg potatoes, peeled and quartered

lots of salt and pepper

5 tablespoons olive oil

1 tablespoon mustard seeds

1 teaspoon ground turmeric

2 teaspoons ground cumin

¼ teaspoon cayenne pepper

juice of 1 lemon

Place the potatoes in a saucepan of cold water, put a lid on the pan and bring to the boil, then add salt. Once the water's boiling, reduce the heat and simmer for 25 minutes, or until they're soft enough to mash.

Meanwhile, heat the oil in a small saucepan over a medium-high heat until it is hot, then add the mustard seeds and wait until they start popping. When this happens, add the rest of the spices, some more salt and pepper, then finally squeeze in the lemon juice and let it bubble for a minute or so. Take it off the heat.

Once the potatoes are cooked, drain them, return them to their hot pan and roughly mash with a fork or wooden spatula; don't let them turn into a mash though, it's nice to keep some chunky texture here.

Stir in the spice mix and devour!

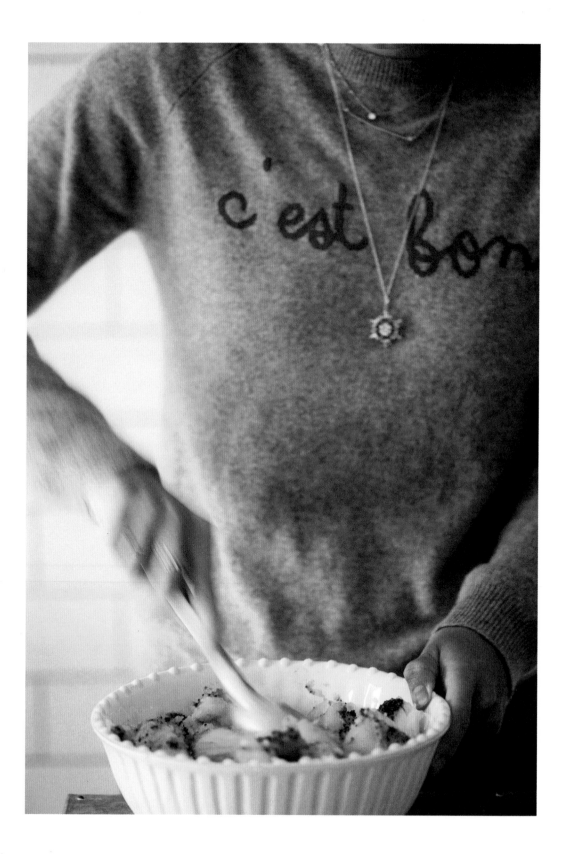

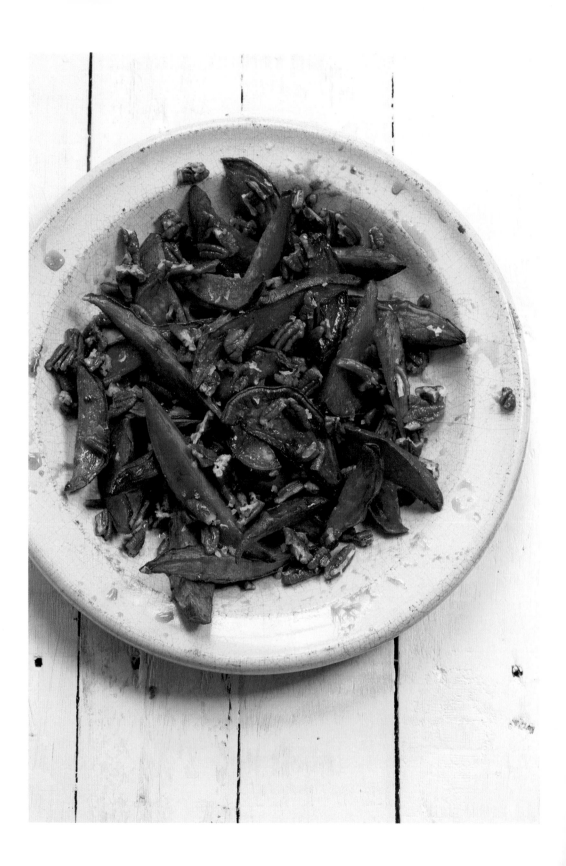

MAPLE & PECAN SWEET POTATOES

These are just a dream. They're always such a crowd-pleaser, so sweet and gooey after they've been baked with maple syrup. If you're trying to convince sceptical friends that veggies are great, then this is your dish. It's simple and totally accessible for everyone.

Serves 4 as a side dish

3 medium sweet potatoes, scrubbed well
    and cut into wedges
2 teaspoons ground cinnamon
2 tablespoons maple syrup
good glug of olive oil
salt and pepper
75g pecans, broken into halves or quarters,
    depending on size

Preheat the oven to 200°C (fan 180°C).

Put the sweet potato wedges on to a baking tray, add the cinnamon, 1 tablespoon of the maple syrup, the olive oil, salt and pepper and mix well with your hands so all the wedges are coated in the mix.

Put in the oven and cook for 40–45 minutes, at which point they should be really tender. Check every so often and turn the wedges halfway through.

Meanwhile, in a small bowl, mix the pecans with the remaining 1 tablespoon of maple syrup, then add them to the sweet potato wedges.

Put the tray back in the oven and let the sweet potatoes and pecans bake together for another 10–15 minutes, until the nuts are golden and crunchy and the sweet potatoes soft and gooey.

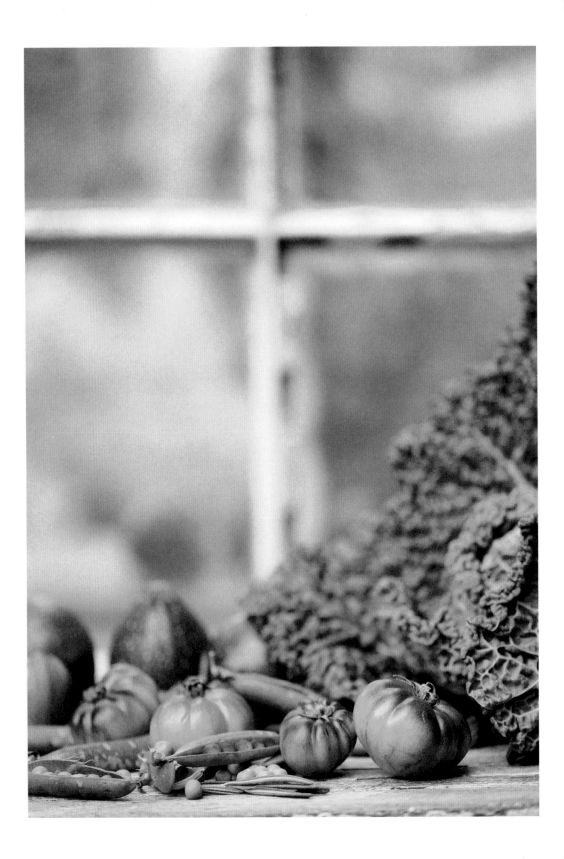

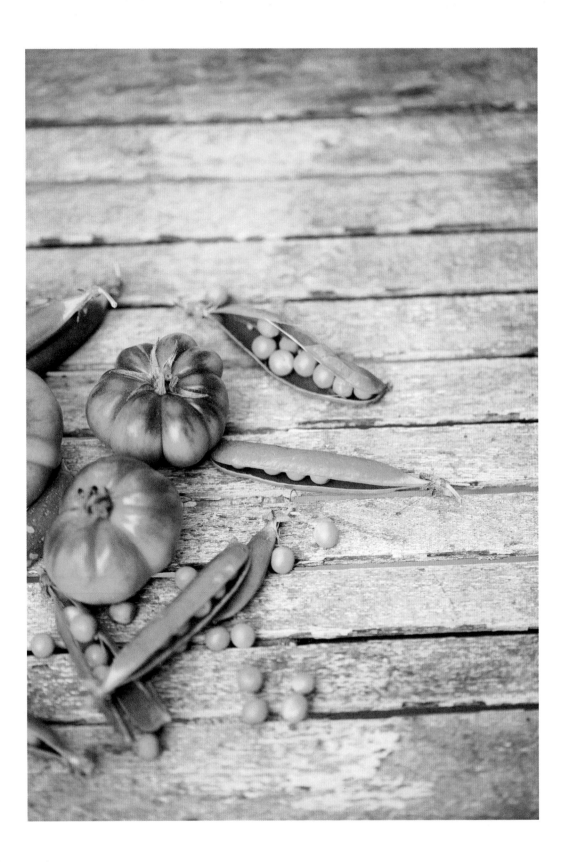

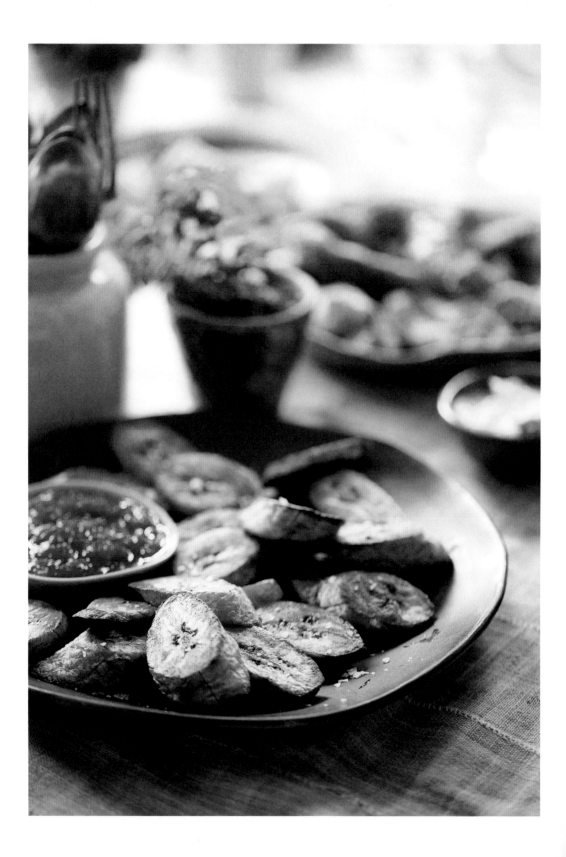

BAKED PLANTAINS WITH SWEET CHILLI SAUCE

*I've become totally obsessed with plantains recently, and they're now one of my absolute
favourite foods. I love them simply baked until golden brown and tender with a little salt,
but they are even better when drizzled with my sweet chilli sauce. The two really work
well together, heightening each other's natural sweetness. I've been serving these with
just about everything lately, from my Sesame Slaw and Pistachio & Apricot Quinoa to
My Favourite Curried Veggies (pages 99, 96 and 150).*

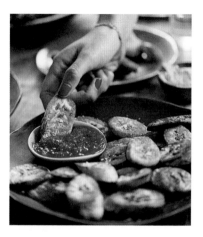

Serves 4

NUT-FREE

FOR THE PLANTAINS
4 plantains
olive oil
salt

FOR THE SWEET CHILLI SAUCE
1 red chilli, deseeded
2.5cm root ginger, peeled and chopped
2 garlic cloves, halved
juice of ½ lime
120ml honey
1 tablespoon apple cider vinegar
salt and pepper
1 teaspoon chia seeds

Preheat the oven to 200°C (fan 180°C).
Peel the plantains and cut into generous
1cm-thick slices. Place in a single layer on
a baking tray. Drizzle with oil and sprinkle
with salt, toss with your hands, then bake
for 50 minutes to 1 hour, until golden brown,
soft and tender. The longer they bake, the
sweeter they get.

Meanwhile, make the sweet chilli sauce.
Put the chilli, ginger and garlic into a food
processor and blitz until finely chopped.

Squeeze the lime juice into a saucepan and
add the honey, vinegar, salt and pepper.
Place over a medium heat, then add the chilli
mixture. Bring to the boil, then add the chia.
Leave to simmer for about 15 minutes until it
thickens. Once thickened, add 2 tablespoons
of water, remove from the heat, scrape into a
small bowl and leave to cool.

Either serve the plantains hot straight from
the oven, or wait for them to cool and serve
them at room temperature. Either way, offer
lots of the sweet chilli sauce on the side.

CLEVER COOKING
While plantains aren't available in every
supermarket, they're generally easy to find
(and often cheaper) in street markets.

SPICY BAKED AVOCADO FRIES WITH A LIME, CASHEW & CORIANDER DIP

These are an absolute revelation, my new favourite way to eat avocados and make a nice change from sweet potato fries. I love the contrast of the soft, creamy chunks of avocado in the middle and the crispy, crunchy, chilli coating on the outside. They're delicious dunked into this lime, cashew and coriander dip too, or, if you want a spicy hit, try the Sweet Chilli Sauce from the plantains (page 187), which tastes amazing with these, too.

Serves 4 as a side dish

FOR THE FRIES

35g gram (chickpea) flour
50ml almond milk, or any other
   plant-based milk
1 tablespoon toasted sesame oil
110g ground almonds
35g sesame seeds
¼ teaspoon cayenne pepper
½ teaspoon salt
¼ teaspoon ground black pepper
½ teaspoon paprika
2 tablespoons nutritional yeast
¼ teaspoon chilli powder
1 teaspoon chilli flakes
2 avocados, ripe but still firm

FOR THE DIP

80g cashew nuts (soaked for 3 hours)
juice of 2½ limes
small handful of fresh coriander (about 8g)
2 tablespoons olive oil
1 tablespoon apple cider vinegar
2 sprigs of fresh mint, leaves picked
pinch of salt

Preheat the oven to 220°C (fan 200°C). Line a baking tray with baking parchment.

Place the gram flour in a bowl. Mix the almond milk and sesame oil in another bowl. Place the ground almonds, sesame seeds, cayenne pepper, salt, pepper, paprika, nutritional yeast and both types of chilli into a third bowl and mix together.

Halve the avocados lengthways, pit and peel, then slice thickly lengthways, making about 5 slices for each avocado half.

Dip the first avocado slice in the gram flour, making sure it's covered. Then dip it in the milk bowl, followed by the ground almonds bowl. Place the coated avocado slice on to the prepared baking tray and repeat for the rest of the avocado slices.

Bake for 20 minutes, flipping halfway through.

Once the avocados are done, remove from the oven. Leave to cool for about 20 minutes; this helps them crisp up even more.

Meanwhile, make the dip. Drain the cashews and tip into a blender. Add 4 tablespoons of water and all the other dip ingredients. Blend until really smooth. Then dip your avocado fries into the sauce and enjoy!

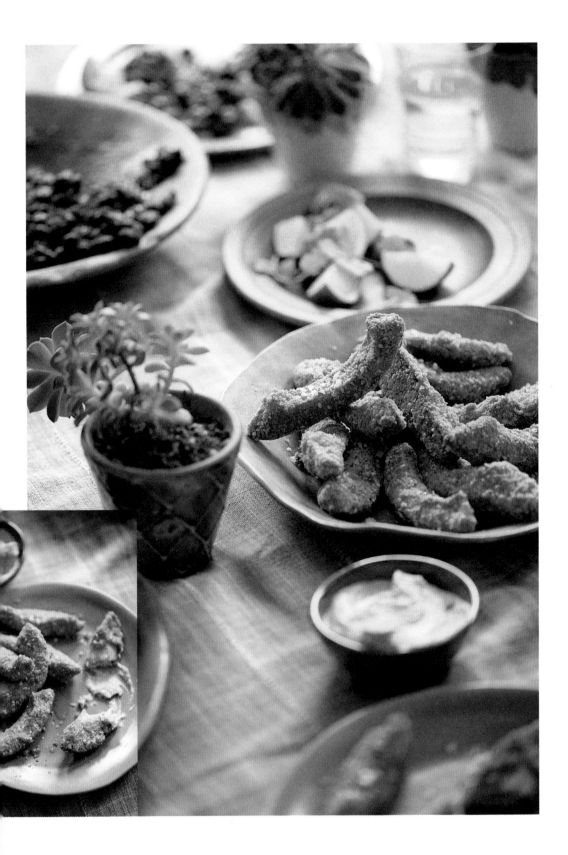

GARLICKY BLACK BEANS

These are a real staple in my diet. I find myself making them all the time as they're quick, cheap and black beans are easy to get hold of. Plus they're a simple way to add a deep, rich flavour to any meal, while also making it feel heartier and more filling. I love them served with simple suppers such as brown rice and mashed avocado when I'm feeling lazy, or as a side for something a little fancier when I'm trying to impress!

Serves 4 as a side dish

NUT-FREE

5 garlic cloves, crushed

2 tablespoons olive oil

¼ teaspoon cayenne pepper

juice of 1 lemon

salt and pepper

2 x 400g cans of black beans,
    drained and rinsed

3 teaspoons brown rice miso paste

3 teaspoons tomato purée

Place the garlic in a saucepan with the olive oil, cayenne pepper, lemon juice and salt and pepper. Gently heat for a minute or so until it starts bubbling.

Add all the other ingredients and cook over a medium heat for about 10 minutes, stirring every couple of minutes. You want the beans to be slightly softened and broken up and fully coated in the miso and tomato purée.

PAN TO PLATE
15 minutes

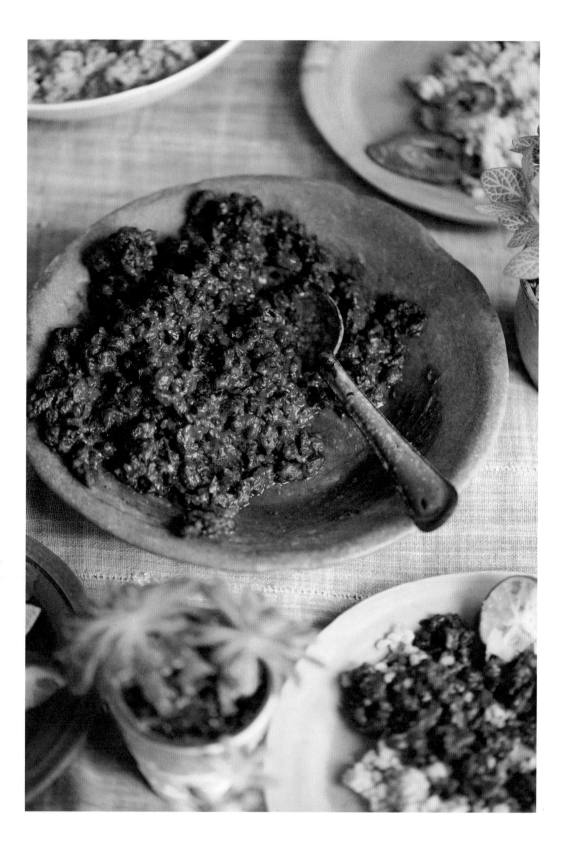

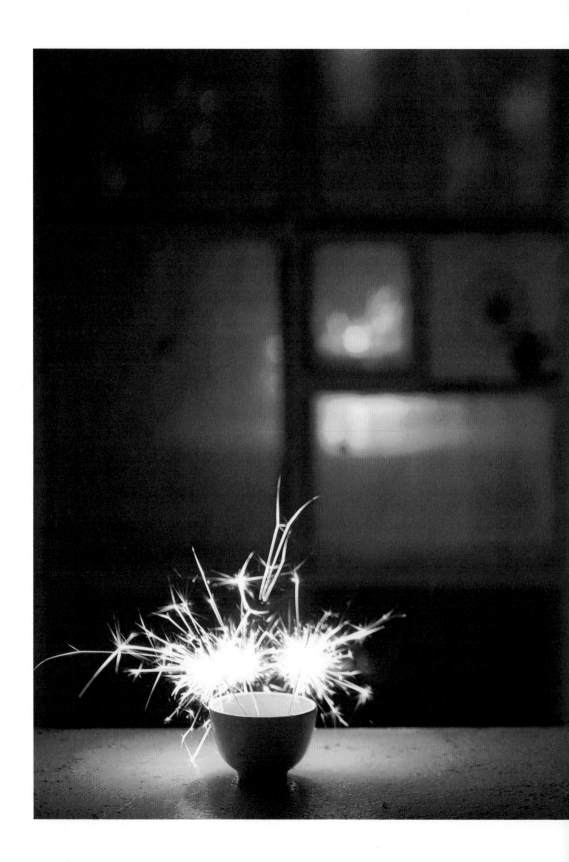

PARTIES

FUN WAYS TO SHARE YOUR FAVOURITE FOODS
WITH THE PEOPLE YOU LOVE

PARTIES

Being kind to yourself with the food you eat doesn't mean that you can't have a lot of fun, and parties are absolutely not ruled out, in fact they're encouraged! You can love yourself, love your food and still have the best time with friends and family. There are so many favourites in the next few pages and it's so hard to single a few things out, but I find myself making the Beet & Sweet Potato Crisps and Smoky Baked Tortilla Chips with big bowls of Smoky Babaganoush and Roast Carrot Hummus for dunking a lot. I also have the best memories of the Watermelon & Cucumber Cooler, that we served at our wedding, and of course nothing can beat a three-tiered Celebration Cake served alongside Blueberry Scones with Vanilla Coconut Cream, or a Banana & Raisin Cake!

MENUS

NIBBLES

Beet & Sweet Potato Crisps

Smoky Baked Tortilla Chips

Roast Carrot Hummus

Smoky Babaganoush

Socca Pizza Bites

Aubergine & Tomato Pesto Rolls with Coconut Tzatziki

Mini Baked Potatoes with Cashew Sour Cream & Chives

Charred Padrón Peppers with Cashew Chipotle Cream

MOCKTAILS & COCKTAILS

Sparkling Pineapple & Cayenne

Coconut, Raspberry & Mint Refresher

Watermelon & Cucumber Cooler

Passion Fruit Spritz

EASY AFTERNOON TEA

Cucumber & Lemon Butter Bean Hummus Open Sandwiches

Banana & Raisin Cake

Ginger Muffins

BIRTHDAY TEA

Peanut Butter & Honey Flapjacks

Celebration Cake

Blueberry Scones with Vanilla Coconut Cream

BEET & SWEET POTATO CRISPS

I love these. They are the most moreish little snacks and they look so beautiful, too, with their bright pink and orange colouring. They taste amazing on their own with just a sprinkling of sea salt, but they're also amazing dunked into Roast Carrot Hummus or Herby Guacamole (pages 200 and 52).

Serves 2

NUT-FREE

1 medium sweet potato, well scrubbed
2 small beetroots, well scrubbed
olive oil
salt

Preheat the oven to 145°C (fan 125°C).

Using a mandolin or a very sharp knife, thinly slice the veg into rounds and lay the slices on to a piece of kitchen paper, then press another piece of kitchen paper over the top to blot them dry.

Lightly brush a couple of baking trays with olive oil, then lay the veg slices on top, making sure they don't overlap or touch. Then pour some more oil into a small bowl and, using a pastry brush, brush oil on to each round. (This step is laborious, but it will make them so crispy and delicious in the end that it's worth taking the time to do it properly. Enjoy the moment!)

Put them in the oven and set the timer for 15 minutes. When the timer goes off, take out each tray, and any that have crisped up nicely can be carefully plucked off and laid onto a wire rack to cool. Turn the rest over on to their other sides, return them to the oven and set the timer for another 10 minutes.

When the timer goes off again, check your trays, and again place any that are done on to the wire rack. The rest go back into the oven for another 5 minutes. When this time is up, they should all be ready, but if not keep going – checking and turning every 5 minutes – until you're satisfied.

Once your crisps are all on the rack and cool, put them in a bowl and sprinkle with a little salt before serving.

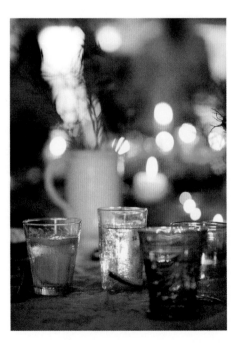

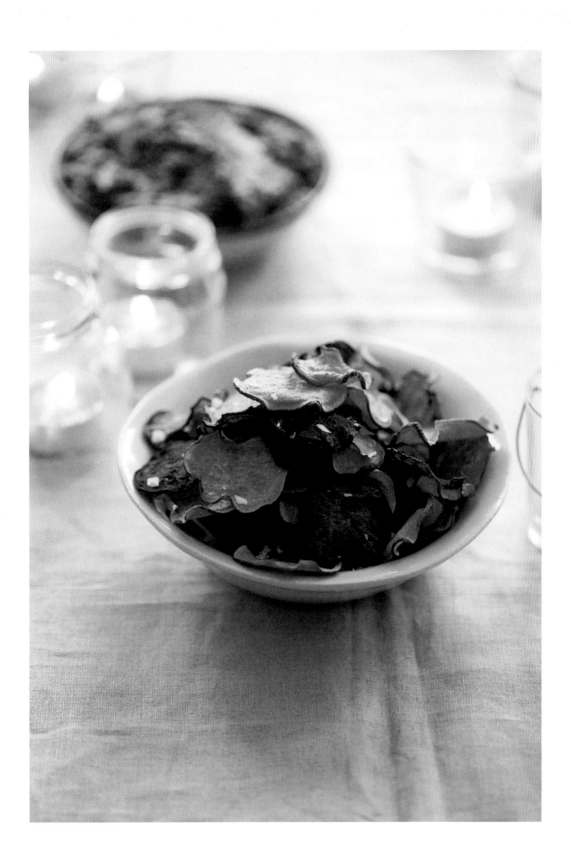

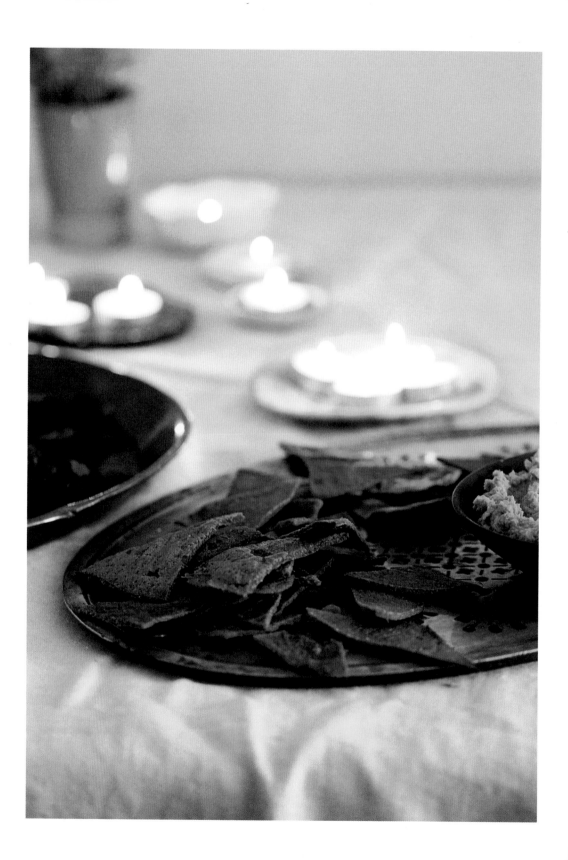

SMOKY BAKED TORTILLA CHIPS

A fantastic addition to any party, these are relatively quick to make, and it's really fun to serve home-made tortilla chips; I'm sure all your friends will be suitably impressed! Perfect with Roast Carrot Hummus (page 200), or any other dip. Be warned, they're addictive, so you may find the whole bowl is gone before your guests even arrive…

Serves 6–8

NUT-FREE

100g buckwheat flour

100g polenta

20g milled (ground) chia seeds (if you can't find them ground, just grind the seeds yourself at home)

1 teaspoon salt

2 heaped teaspoons smoked paprika

2 teaspoons chilli flakes

1 teaspoon honey

Preheat the oven to 200°C (fan 180°C).

Mix all the dry ingredients in a bowl. Add the honey, then pour in 150ml of water. Mix into a paste with a fork and set aside.

On a clean dry surface, lay down a square of baking parchment. Cut another square of baking parchment and set aside.

Wet your hands and pick up half the tortilla mix from the bowl. Roll it in your palms until it's a nice smooth ball and drop it into the centre of the baking parchment. Place the second sheet of baking parchment on top and squash the dough down gently with your hand into a disc. Take a rolling pin and roll it from the centre outwards to make a nice circle, about 20cm across. Place on a baking sheet, leaving both sheets of baking parchment on. Repeat to roll the remaining dough and place on a separate baking sheet.

Put both tortillas in the oven for 10 minutes, then remove and peel off the top layers of baking parchment. Cut into 8 pieces, as you would cut a pizza. (You can use a knife, but I find scissors much easier.) The tortilla will be hot, so watch you don't burn your fingers, but do it straight away or it will become too brittle to cut. Repeat with the second tortilla.

Return the tortilla triangles to their baking sheets and bake for 5 minutes until they harden up. Cool on a wire rack, then serve as soon as possible.

ROAST CARROT HUMMUS

As lots of you will know by now, hummus is one of my favourite foods, and I find that all my friends and family love it, too. Everyone always gets so excited by how much better home-made hummus tastes than the shop-bought versions! I make a variety of hummus almost every time I have people over, as it's such a good pre-dinner snack, and it's so easy to throw together in no time. I especially love this carroty one, as the colour is so fantastic. Once I've made my hummus, I just scoop it out of the food processor into a nice bowl and lay it out with my Smoky Baked Tortilla Chips (page 199) for everyone to enjoy when they arrive. If I want it to look more impressive, I'll drizzle it with a little olive oil, then sprinkle toasted pine nuts and smoked paprika over the top.

Makes 1 bowl

NUT-FREE

4 medium carrots (about 400g), peeled

1½ teaspoons paprika

10 tablespoons olive oil, plus more
    for the carrots

salt

3 garlic cloves, peeled

2 x 400g cans of chickpeas, drained
    and rinsed

3 tablespoons tahini

juice of 2 juicy lemons, or 3 if they're not
    very juicy

1 teaspoon ground cumin

Preheat the oven to 220°C (fan 200°C).

Chop the carrots into quarters, then put them on a baking tray with ½ teaspoon of the paprika, a drizzle of olive oil and a sprinkling of salt. Roast for about 40 minutes, until soft and tender, adding the garlic cloves for the last 10 minutes. Leave to cool.

Meanwhile, place the chickpeas into a food processor with the 10 tablespoons of olive oil, the tahini, lemon juice, remaining 1 teaspoon of paprika, the ground cumin and salt, spoon in 4 tablespoons of water and blend until smooth and creamy.

Once the carrots and garlic have cooled, add them to the processor and finish blending. When the hummus is smooth and creamy, scoop it into a bowl and serve.

This will keep in an airtight container in the fridge for up to 7 days.

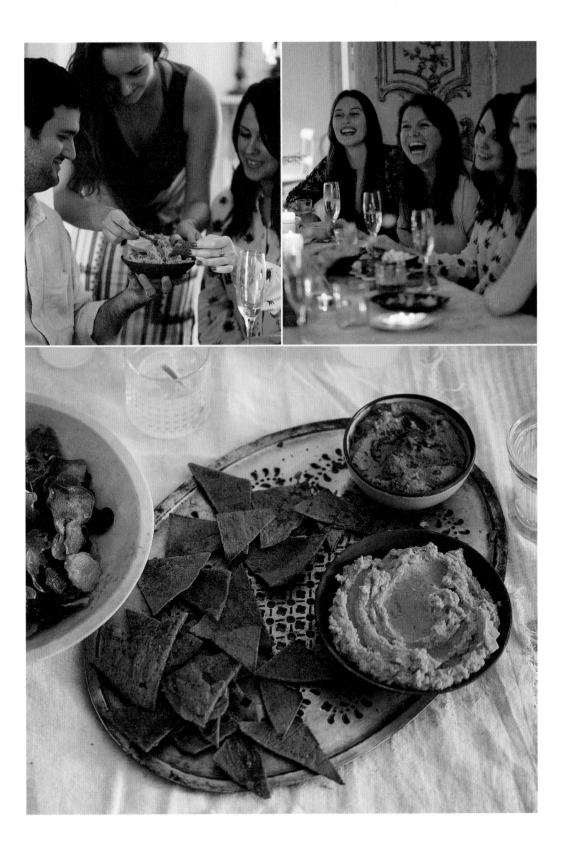

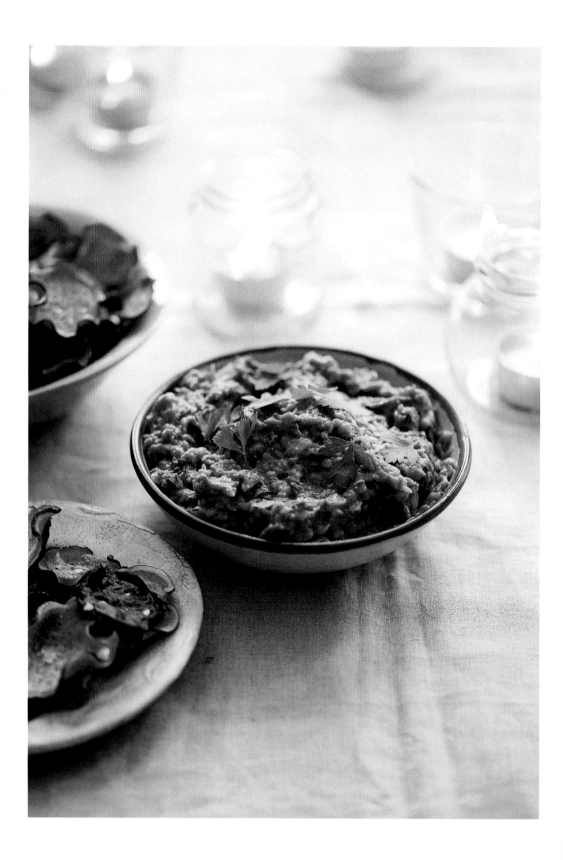

SMOKY BABAGANOUSH

One of my best-loved dips; I just love how rich and creamy this is. Chunky baked aubergine adds such a great texture, while the paprika and cayenne really liven it up and add a smoky spice to each bite. I like to serve this to friends with Smoky Baked Tortilla Chips (page 199) or crackers as a pre-lunch snack, or just to dollop it on the side of a grain and veggie bowl.

Makes 1 big bowl

NUT-FREE

3 aubergines
1 bulb of garlic
3 tablespoons olive oil, plus more to roast
   the aubergine and garlic
juice of 1 lemon
1 tablespoon tahini
2 teaspoons smoked paprika
½ teaspoon ground cumin
¼ teaspoon cayenne pepper
salt and pepper
handful of fresh parsley leaves,
   roughly chopped

Preheat the oven to 220°C (fan 200°C).

Prick each aubergine in a couple of places with a knife; this is essential to stop them from exploding as they bake! Put them on a baking tray and bake for 40 minutes, turning halfway through. Place the whole bulb of garlic, just as it is, in a square of foil, drizzle with oil, then seal the foil as though it was a little parcel (this stops it burning) and pop it into the baking tray in the oven alongside the aubergines for 30 minutes.

After the aubergines have cooked for 40 minutes, their skins should be blackened and the insides feel soft when pressed. Take the aubergines and garlic out of the oven, cut the aubergines in half lengthways and leave everything to cool.

When they're cool enough to handle, scoop out the flesh of the aubergines, and squeeze out the sticky sweet baked garlic from its cloves. Add the aubergine flesh and garlic to a blender, then add all the other ingredients except the parsley (not forgetting the 3 tablespoons of oil) and pulse a few times rather than blending completely, to avoid a totally smooth purée; you want some nice texture in there. Stir in the parsley and eat!

SOCCA PIZZA BITES

The perfect little canapé. They're so easy to make and only need a couple of really simple ingredients, plus they look fantastic. I love serving them with a dollop of the sun-dried tomato pesto below, a few chopped black olives, a sprinkling of wild rocket and a drizzle of olive oil, to heighten all the flavours. Socca is a French / Italian flatbread or pancake made from chickpea flour, and utterly addictive.

Makes about 24

NUT-FREE

FOR THE PESTO

60g sun-dried tomatoes in oil
   (drained weight)

25g pine nuts

15g fresh basil

2 tablespoons olive oil

1 garlic clove, roughly chopped

salt and pepper

½ tablespoon apple cider vinegar

FOR THE PIZZAS

100g gram (chickpea) flour

2 teaspoons mixed dried herbs

drizzle of olive oil

chopped black olives, to serve

wild rocket leaves, to serve

First make the pesto by blending all the ingredients together with 2 tablespoons of water in a food processer until a chunky paste forms.

In a mixing bowl whisk together the chickpea flour and mixed herbs with 150ml of water, seasoning to taste, until a totally smooth batter forms, Leave to sit for 30 minutes so the flour can totally absorb the water.

Once you're ready to make the pizzas, heat a drizzle of olive oil in a frying pan and, when it's hot, spoon in 1 teaspoon of the batter at a time to make each mini pizza.

Cook over a medium heat for 1–2 minutes, then flip and cook for another 1–2 minutes on the other side, until golden brown. Repeat this process until you have cooked all the pizza bites.

Spoon the pesto on to the pizza bases and top with the olives and a few rocket leaves to serve.

CLEVER COOKING

Try to serve these while they're still warm, as they taste even better!

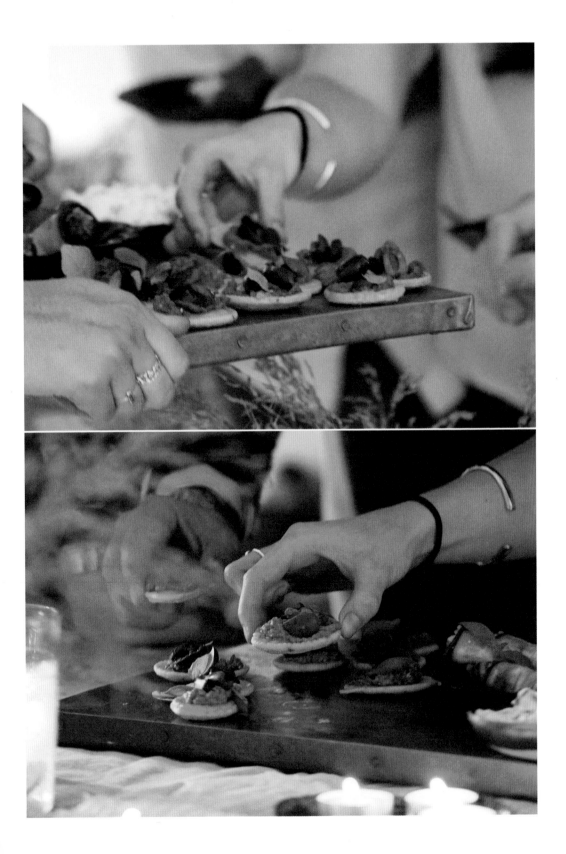

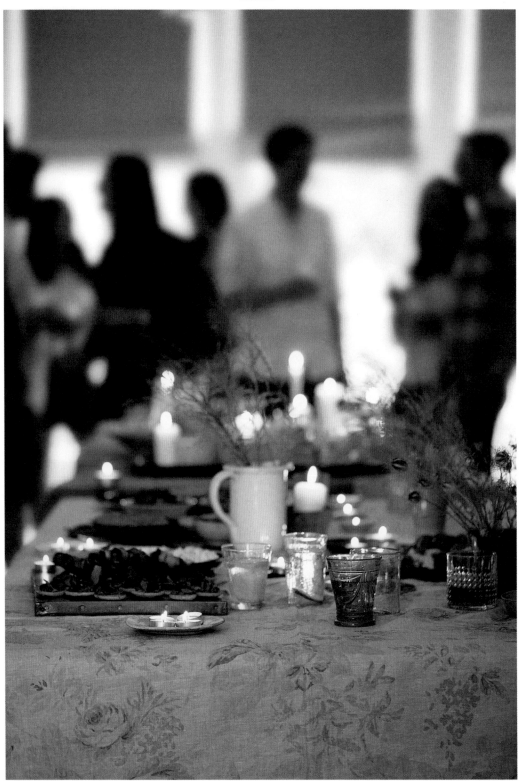

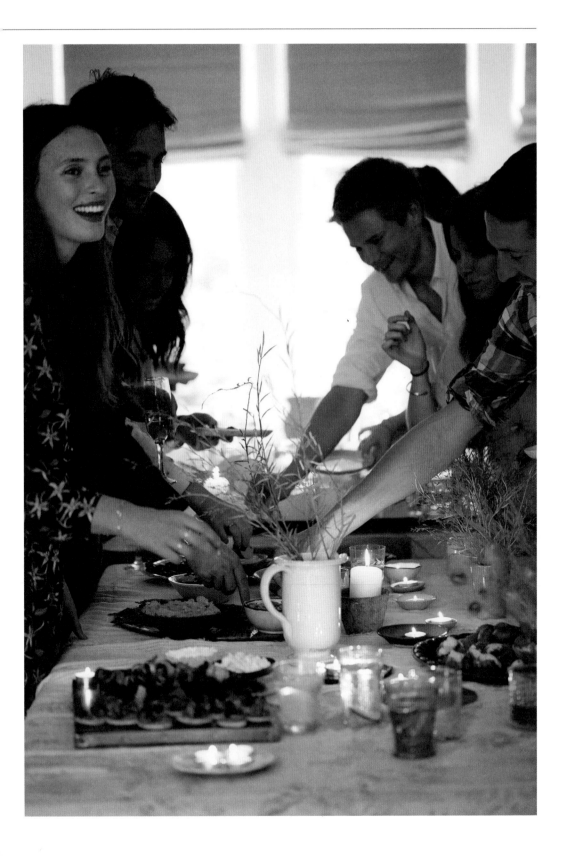

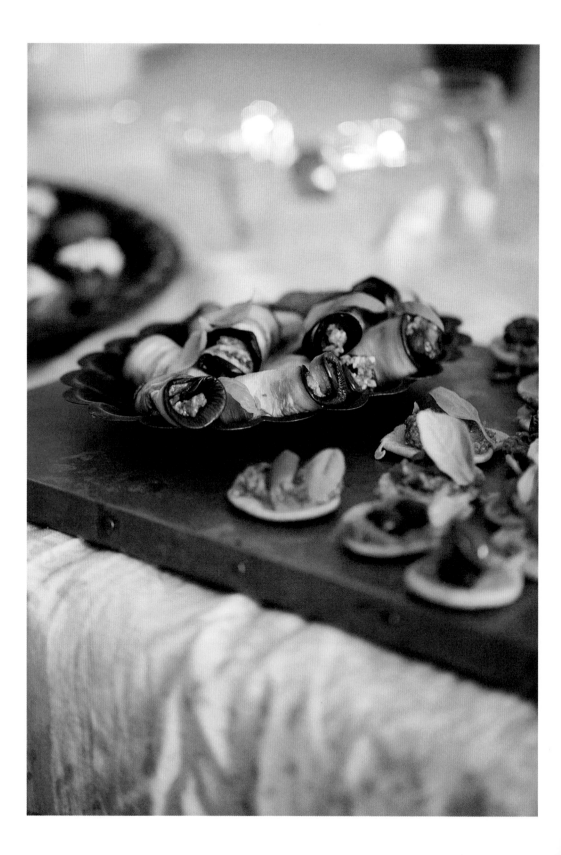

AUBERGINE & TOMATO PESTO ROLLS WITH COCONUT TZATZIKI

So great on their own, but when these rolls are dunked into the creamy mint and cucumber yogurt dip here, they become something truly special. The contrast of the hot rolls against the smooth cool dip is really amazing. These are definitely among the recipes I recommend you try first from this book; it's one of the best! The pesto is essentially the same as for Socca Pizza Bites (page 204), sharpened with lemon juice.

Makes 15 bite-sized rolls

NUT-FREE

FOR THE AUBERGINES
2 large aubergines
2 tablespoons olive oil
salt and pepper

FOR THE PESTO
40g pine nuts
280g jar of sun-dried tomatoes in oil, drained (170g drained weight)
small handful of fresh basil
1 small garlic clove
juice of ½ lemon

FOR THE DIP
½ cucumber
leaves from a few sprigs of fresh mint
250g coconut yogurt
juice of 1 lemon

CLEVER COOK

These work really well with a classic pesto, too, so if you're tight on time or don't have a food processor to blend the pesto in, you can always buy a jar and stuff the rolls with that.

Preheat the oven to 220°C (fan 200°C).

Slice the aubergines thinly lengthways (use a sharp knife). Drizzle a couple of large baking trays with the olive oil and a sprinkling of salt, lay the aubergine slices evenly across them and place in the oven. Cook for about 20 minutes, until soft and tender enough to roll.

Meanwhile, make the pesto. Simply place all the ingredients in a food processor and blitz until they form a chunky paste.

Let the aubergine slices cool for a few minutes, then cut each in half widthways. Put 1 heaped teaspoon of pesto at the top of each, then roll them up. (You can use cocktail sticks to keep them together if you want.)

To make the dipping sauce, deseed the cucumber by halving it lengthways and running a teaspoon along the centre. Cut it into little cubes (about 5mm). Finely chop the mint. Place the mint and cucumber in a bowl with the yogurt and lemon juice, season to taste and stir. Serve with the aubergine rolls.

MINI BAKED POTATOES WITH CASHEW SOUR CREAM & CHIVES

An amazing little nibble for hungry friends. These warm, salt-crusted potatoes are stuffed with a creamy cashew sour cream, then sprinkled with lots of black pepper, chives and fresh chilli to make something incredibly delicious. They're perfect in the winter, hearty and comforting, and will keep everyone happy while you finish making dinner.

Serves 6

FOR THE POTATOES
500g new potatoes
1 tablespoon olive oil
sea salt flakes and lots of black pepper
1 red chilli

FOR THE CASHEW SOUR CREAM
120g cashew nuts (soaked for 4 hours)
juice of 1½ lemons
1 tablespoon apple cider vinegar
salt and pepper
8g chives, finely chopped
3 spring onions, finely chopped

CLEVER COOKING
Serve these on a warmed tray so that they don't get cold too quickly.

Preheat the oven to 210°C (fan 190°C). Line a baking tray with a sheet of baking parchment.

Prick the skin of the potatoes with a fork, then rub them with the olive oil and sprinkle them with a generous amount of sea salt flakes. Place them on the prepared tray and bake for 1 hour, until crisp on the outside and tender on the inside.

Let them cool for 10–15 minutes, until they're still warm but not boiling. Then, cut a cross in the top of each and squeeze up from the base to open the cut a little (use a tea towel to protect your hands from burning).

While they cool, make the cashew sour cream (for the method, see page 115), adding 2 tablespoons of water as in that recipe, but using only 5g of the chives. Chop the remaining chives and the red chilli (discard the seeds).

Add 1 teaspoon of the cashew sour cream to each potato, pushing it into the opening. Grind lots of black pepper over the top and sprinkle with salt, chives and chilli.

Serve straight away.

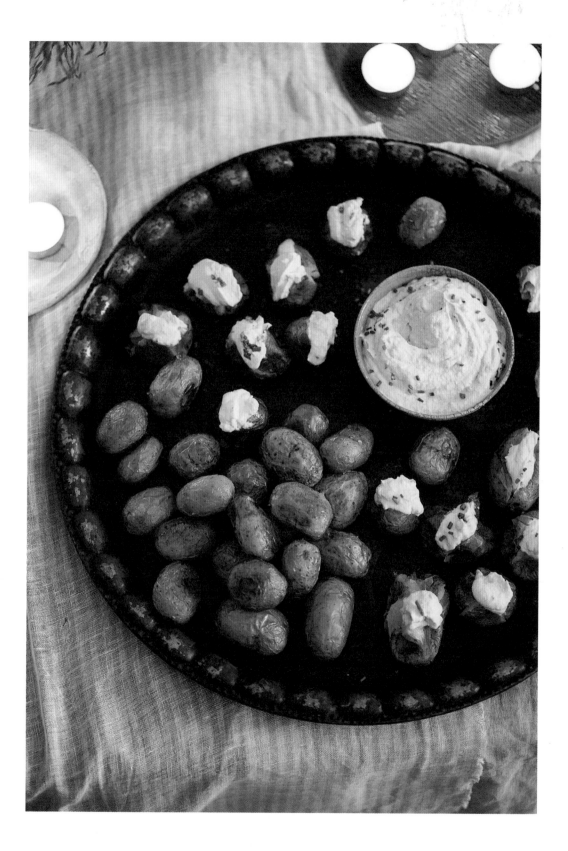

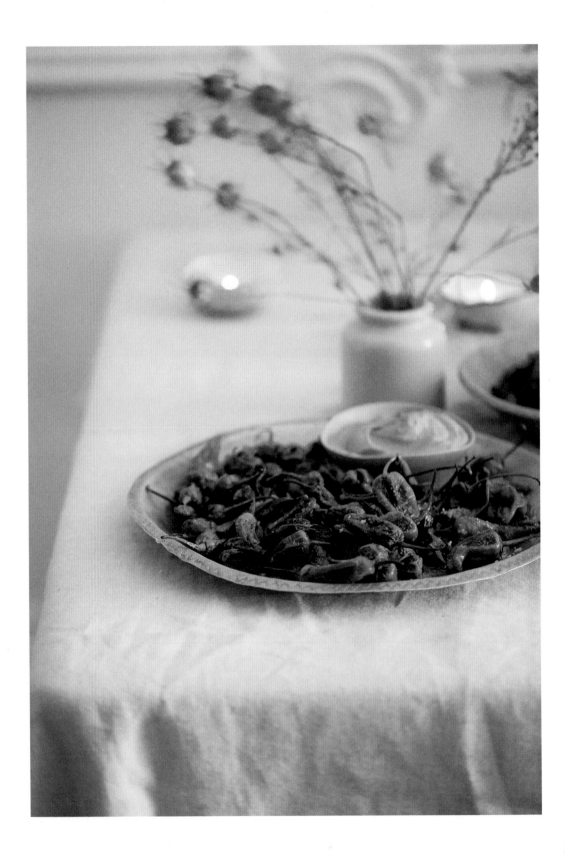

CHARRED PADRÓN PEPPERS WITH CASHEW CHIPOTLE CREAM

Padrón peppers are always one of the first things I look for on a restaurant menu; I just love them. They're so moreish, especially when they're nicely blistered and piping hot. I find they're especially good when you have something to dip them in, which is where this chipotle cream comes in. It's wonderfully smoky, with tangy hints of lemon and deeply savoury sesame oil.

Makes 1 bowl

FOR THE CASHEW CREAM
150g cashews (soaked for 4 hours)
3 tablespoons olive oil
2 teaspoons chipotle powder
½ teaspoon smoked paprika
juice of 2 lemons
2 tablespoons apple cider vinegar
1 teaspoon toasted sesame oil
generous amount of salt

FOR THE PEPPERS
300g padrón peppers
olive oil
sea salt flakes

Drain the soaked cashews, then tip them into a blender and measure in 12 tablespoons of water. Add all the other ingredients for the chipotle cream and blend until the mix is smooth and creamy. Scrape it into a bowl.

Put the peppers in a large frying pan with a little olive oil and a generous amount of sea salt flakes and fry until they start to blister; this should take about 10 minutes.

Serve the peppers with the chipotle cream.

PAN TO PLATE
10 minutes, plus soaking time

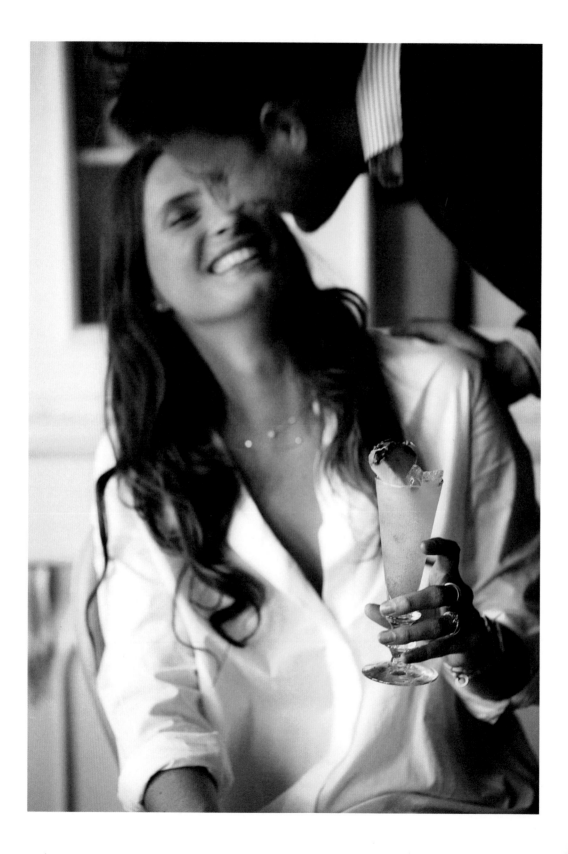

SPARKLING PINEAPPLE & CAYENNE

One of my all-time favourite drinks, this is amazingly sweet and refreshing with a subtle hint of spice from the ginger and cayenne and a little tanginess from lime juice, plus a subtle sparkle from the soda water. I like serving it in short glasses with lots of ice, a wedge of juicy pineapple and a sprinkling of more cayenne... it's the perfect addition to any summer party or dinner with friends. If you want to make these really fun, serve them in carved-out pineapples! You can make this in a juicer or a blender.

Serves 3

NUT-FREE

1 ripe pineapple
2.5cm root ginger, peeled
1 glass of soda water (about 400ml)
juice of ½ lime
2 teaspoons maple syrup
generous pinch of cayenne pepper, to taste
   (I like quite a lot, about 3 pinches), plus
   more to serve
dash of your favourite spirit (optional)
ice cubes

Cut the hard skin off the pineapple, then cut a small slice off the top for garnishing later. Put the rest of the pineapple through a juicer with the ginger, passing the ginger through towards the start of the operation, to get the most flavour out of it.

Pour the juice through a sieve into a jug, to make sure it's really smooth.

Pour the soda water into the jug, then add the lime juice, maple syrup and cayenne to taste, along with the spirit, if you like. Stir well.

Fill 3 short glasses with ice and pour the drink into each. Sprinkle with a pinch more cayenne and add a wedge of pineapple from the reserved slice to the side of the glass.

CLEVER COOKING
If you don't have a juicer, put the ginger and pineapple in your blender instead, then strain the blended mixture through a sieve to make it smooth.

COCONUT, RASPBERRY & MINT REFRESHER

This is a wonderfully refreshing drink made from cooling coconut water, lime juice and maple syrup, stirred with fresh mint, cucumber slices and raspberries. It looks beautiful with the mix of greens and pinks, so a big jug of this is a lovely addition to any table. Measure out the coconut water using the glasses in which you will be serving it.

Serves 3

NUT-FREE

¼ cucumber

25g sprigs of fresh mint

2½ long glasses of coconut water, preferably raw and unpasteurised

juice of 2 limes

2 teaspoons maple syrup

50g raspberries

ice cubes

dash of your favourite spirit (optional)

Thinly slice the cucumber and tear the mint leaves off their stems. Keep the leaves and discard the stems.

Pour the coconut water into a jug with the lime juice and maple syrup. Stir well, then add the cucumber slices, mint leaves and raspberries.

Let the drink sit in the fridge for at least 30 minutes, so that the flavours can be absorbed into the water.

Once you're ready to serve, add ice cubes to 3 glasses and stir your spirit into the jug, if you're using one.

Pour the mix into the glasses, trying to get the mint, cucumber and raspberries evenly distributed between them.

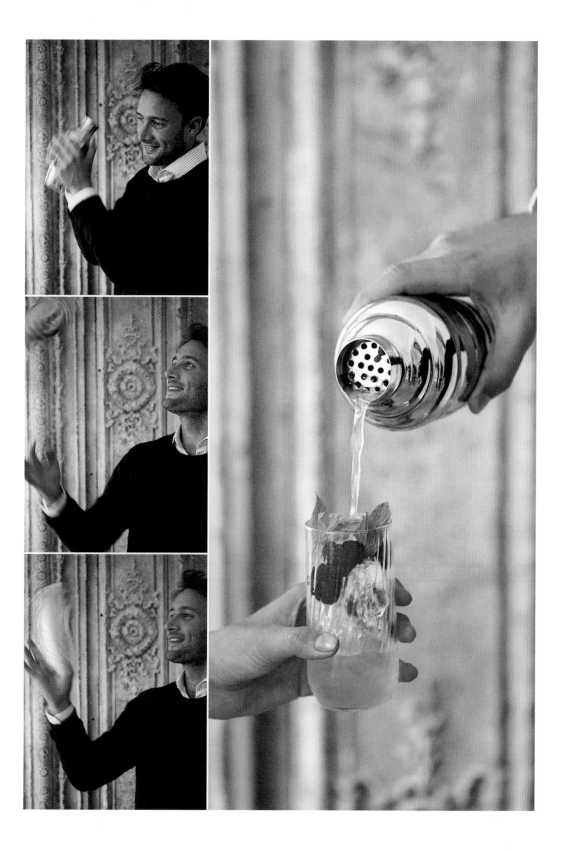

PASSION FRUIT SPRITZ

This is so lovely and I'm sure will be a big hit with all your friends. The tropical mix tastes amazing with a little vanilla powder and sparkling water. Try serving this with the Mexican Fiesta (pages 110–117), they're perfect together.

Serves 2

NUT-FREE

½ mango, peeled and pitted
3 passion fruits, flesh scooped out
½ lime
½ teaspoon vanilla powder
200ml sparkling water
ice cubes

Work the mango and passion fruits through a juicer. Squeeze in the lime juice, then add the vanilla and give it a good stir.

Pour into 2 short glasses, then top up both with sparkling water and a few ice cubes.

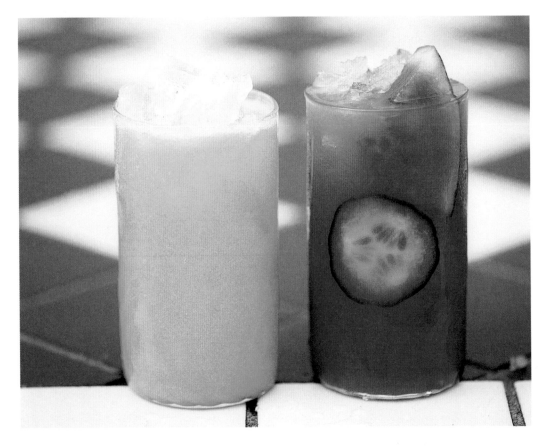

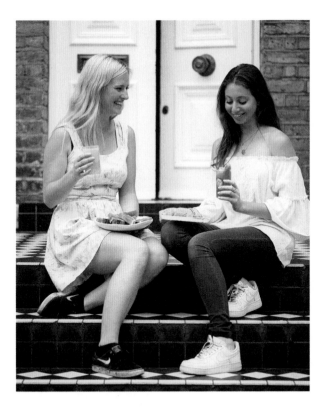

WATERMELON & CUCUMBER COOLER

*This is a great summer drink, sweet and refreshing with a lovely mix of watermelon,
cucumber and strawberries. We served this at our wedding and everyone loved it!
It's simple and quick to make and very unfussy; it just needs five minutes to make, so you
and your guests will have a delicious drink in no time.*

Serves 2

NUT-FREE

½ cucumber

400g watermelon flesh, rind cut off,
  and deseeded

5 strawberries, hulled

2 teaspoons maple syrup (optional)

dash of your favourite spirit (optional)

ice cubes

Juice the cucumber.

Pour the juice into a blender with the
watermelon, strawberries and maple syrup,
if using. Blend until smooth. Pour through a
sieve into a jug to remove any lumps, then
spoon any excess foam off the top.

Stir in the spirit, if using.

Add ice cubes to 2 long glasses and pour
the drink in.

CUCUMBER & LEMON BUTTER BEAN HUMMUS OPEN SANDWICHES

These simple little sandwiches are a lovely addition to any afternoon tea or snack time.
The creamy, lemony hummus tastes amazing topped with crunchy slices of cucumber,
a sprinkling of lemon zest and lots of black pepper. I often make these as an afternoon
snack and keep the rest of the hummus in the fridge to use throughout the week, dolloped
on the side of other meals.

Makes 12

NUT-FREE

FOR THE HUMMUS

400g can of butter beans,
   drained and rinsed
1 tablespoon tahini
juice of 1½ lemons
2 teaspoons ground cumin
2 tablespoons olive oil
1 garlic clove
salt

FOR THE SANDWICHES

3 large slices of square bread
   (I use rye bread)
½ cucumber, thinly sliced
finely grated zest and juice of
   1 unwaxed lemon
sea salt flakes and lots of black pepper

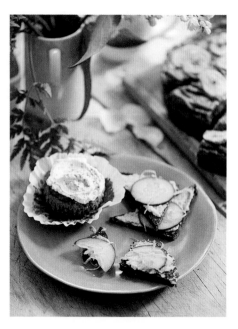

First make the hummus. Simply place everything in a food processor and blend until smooth and creamy.

Either toast the bread, if you want it crunchy, or leave it (I find rye bread and most gluten-free breads are nicer toasted).

Spread a thick layer of hummus over the bread or toast, then add crunchy slices of cucumber. Sprinkle with lemon zest to add colour and texture, then squeeze a little lemon juice on each, sprinkle with sea salt flakes and grind over lots of black pepper. Cut each into quarters to serve.

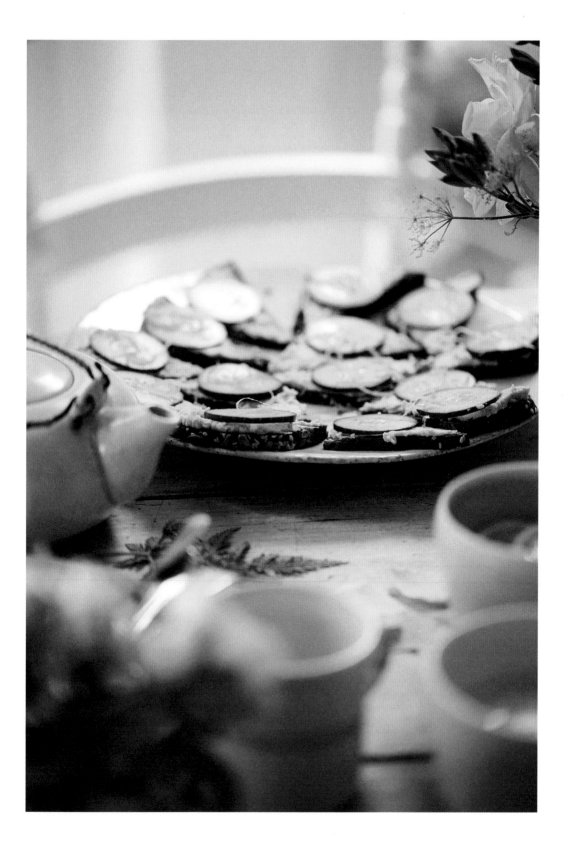

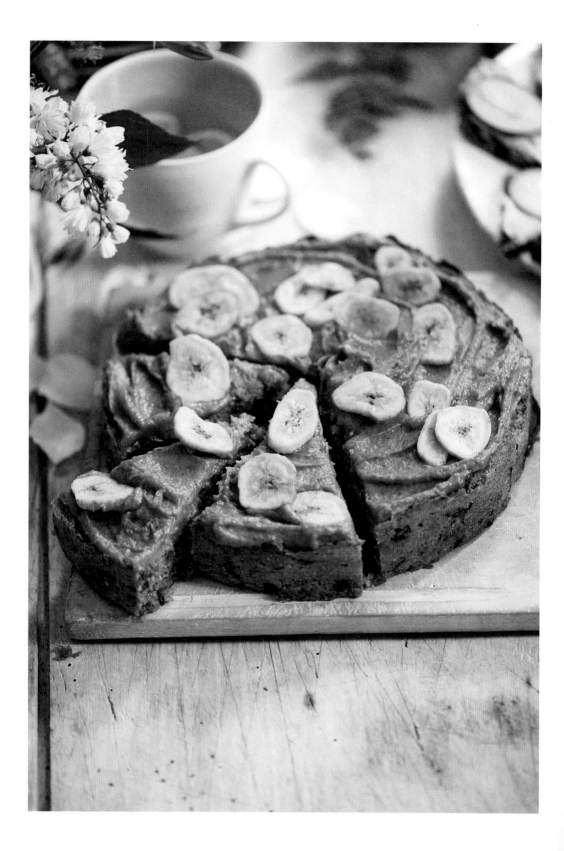

BANANA & RAISIN CAKE

This is one of my favourite cakes; it's such a great treat to serve your friends and family. It's soft and light, with juicy bites of raisins and sweet hints of coconut. It's a pretty easy recipe, plus it's the best way to use up old bananas, which I always seem to have in my kitchen! Your guests will absolutely love feasting on slices of this alongside Ginger Muffins and Cucumber & Lemon Butter Bean Hummus Open Sandwiches (pages 224 and 220); together they make a really wonderful afternoon tea.

Makes 1 cake

FOR THE CAKE

2 tablespoons coconut oil,
  plus more for the tin
4 over-ripe bananas
300g oats
360g Apple Purée (page 23)
3 teaspoons ground cinnamon
2 teaspoons vanilla powder
4 tablespoons coconut sugar
150g raisins
2 tablespoons chia seeds

FOR THE ICING

2 over-ripe bananas, peeled
4 medjool dates, pitted
1 teaspoon vanilla powder
2 tablespoons coconut oil
2 tablespoons almond butter
½ teaspoon ground cinnamon,
  plus more to serve
banana chips, to decorate (optional)

Preheat the oven to 200°C (fan 180°C). Use coconut oil to oil a 22cm diameter round cake tin, or line it with baking parchment.

Peel the bananas for the cake, mash with a fork and put them in a large bowl. Grind the oats into a flour in a food processor. Melt the 2 tablespoons of coconut oil in a small saucepan. Now simply mix all the ingredients together and scrape the batter into the prepared tin.

Bake for 50 minutes, or until a knife poked in comes out clean, then let it cool – still in the tin – for 30 minutes to finish setting.

Meanwhile, make the icing. Simply blend all the ingredients (except the banana chips) until totally smooth, then put the icing in the fridge to set for 10–20 minutes, while the cake cools.

When the cake is totally cool, remove it from the tin and spread the icing over the top. Decorate with banana chips, if you like, and sprinkle with cinnamon.

GINGER MUFFINS

I'm a big ginger fan. I love the warming sensation it brings to any dish, especially when combined with vanilla, cinnamon and nutmeg, as it is here. The spices work so well in this muffin, creating a really uplifting little afternoon snack. The icing is totally optional, if you want something that's easy to carry around then I'd skip it as it can get messy in a lunch box, but if you're staying put then absolutely add it, as it heightens the deliciousness and adds a smooth, creamy texture to the oaty muffin.

Makes 12

NUT-FREE

FOR THE MUFFINS

250g coconut yogurt

2 tablespoons psyllium husk (from health
food shops or online)

175g brown rice flour

50g coconut flour

70g oats

100g coconut sugar

2 teaspoons ground cinnamon,
plus more to serve (optional)

2 teaspoons vanilla powder

1 teaspoon ground nutmeg

3 teaspoons ground ginger,
plus more to serve (optional)

2 over-ripe bananas, peeled and mashed

2 tablespoons coconut oil, melted

2 tablespoons maple syrup

FOR THE ICING

250g coconut yogurt

1 teaspoon ground ginger

2 tablespoons maple syrup

Preheat the oven to 200°C (fan 180°C) and place 12 muffin cases into a muffin tin.

Make the muffin batter. Pour the coconut yogurt into a large bowl. Make a psyllium husk 'egg' (this helps the batter to stick together): place the husk in a small bowl or mug with 4 tablespoons of water and give it a mix. Pour into the coconut yogurt and whisk thoroughly to combine.

Add the dry ingredients, then stir in 150ml of water. Stir in the bananas, coconut oil and maple syrup and mix until it forms quite a stiff batter. Spoon the batter evenly between the muffin cases.

Bake for 40 minutes. Let cool completely in the tin before icing (or the icing will melt).

To make the icing, simply mix all the ingredients together in a bowl and let it sit in the fridge for the last few minutes of the muffins cooling.

Ice each muffin and sprinkle with ground ginger or cinnamon before serving, if you like.

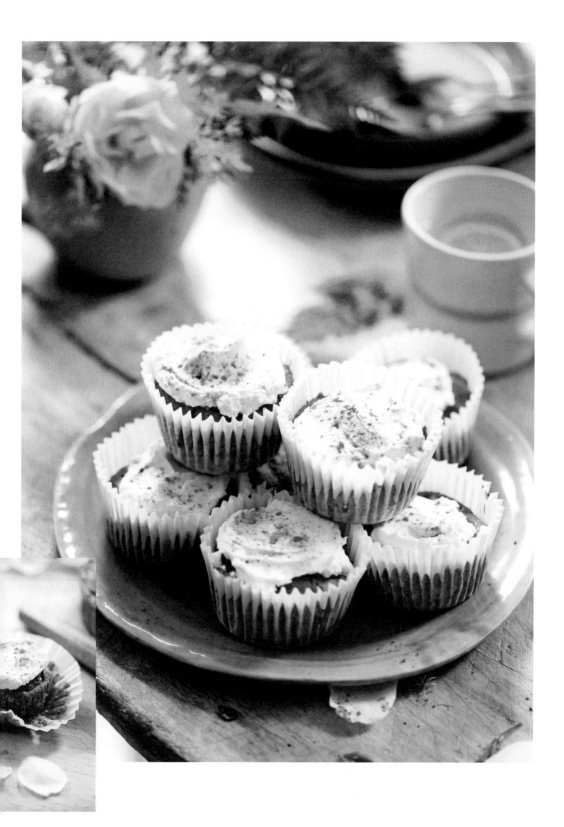

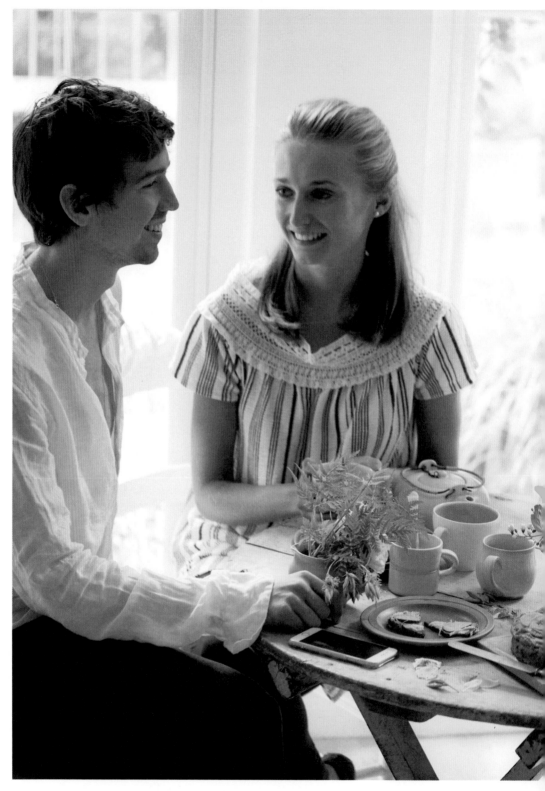

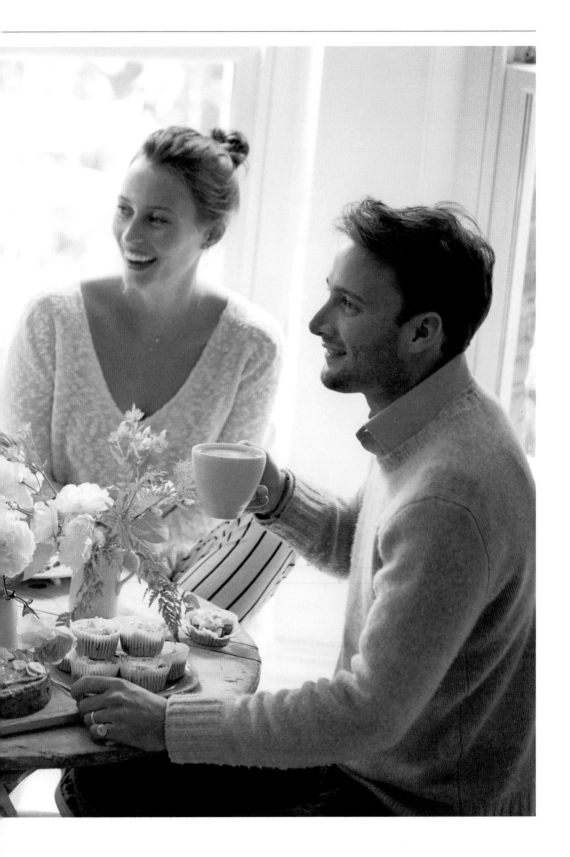

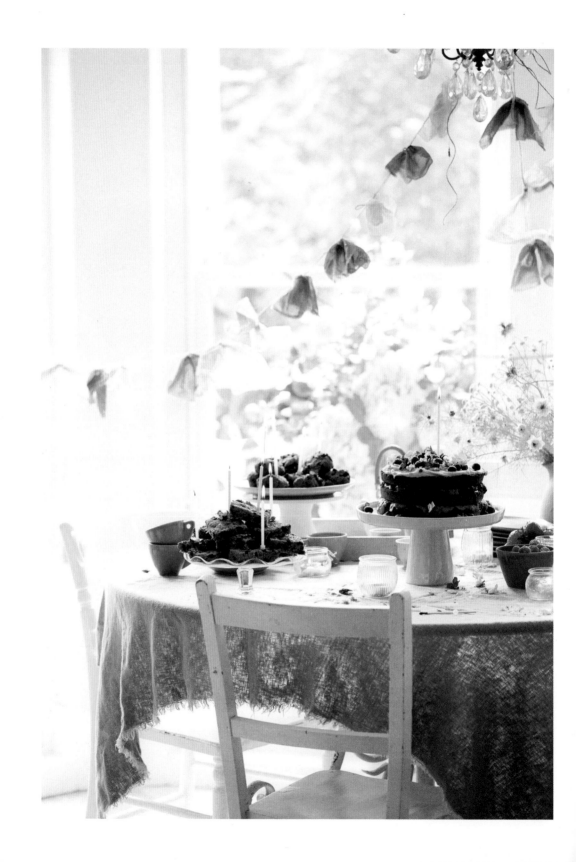

PEANUT BUTTER & HONEY FLAPJACKS

These are so moreish; I always get through a batch of them far too quickly! The mix of banana and peanut butter makes each bite soft and gooey, while the raisins, coconut oil and honey give a deliciously sweet taste, although, as there's only four spoons of honey across the whole batch, they're not overly sweet, which means they also work really well as an on-the-go breakfast.

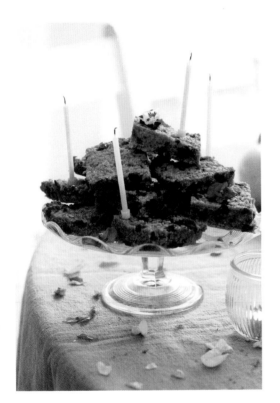

Makes 12

4 over-ripe bananas
4 tablespoons honey
4 tablespoons crunchy peanut butter,
   or any other nut butter
200g raisins
300g oats
3 tablespoons coconut oil, plus more
   for the tin

Preheat the oven to 200°C (fan 180°C).

Peel the bananas, place in a bowl and mash them with a fork. Mix in all the other ingredients.

Oil a 20cm square brownie tin with coconut oil, or line with baking parchment, and pour the mix into the prepared tin.

Bake for 30–35 minutes, until golden brown. Then take the tray out the oven and let it sit for at least 15 minutes for the flapjacks to finish setting. Once they're cool, cut into 12 bars and enjoy!

CELEBRATION CAKE

If you've got a birthday or a special event coming up that needs a sweet, indulgent cake to mark it, then this is for you. It looks incredibly impressive and decadent with its layers of vanilla and almond sponge layered with blueberry jam and caramel icing, then finished with coconut icing on top. The triple-layered effect makes it visually stunning, while the three different icings mean it's delicious. I tend to always go for chocolatey cakes, so this is a really nice change, and losing the chocolate also makes it feel a little lighter, so you can enjoy an extra few bites... or even another slice!

Serves 8–10

FOR THE CAKE

4½ tablespoons coconut oil, plus more
    for the tins
3 tablespoons chia seeds
2 teaspoons apple cider vinegar
360ml almond milk
360ml maple syrup
9 teaspoons vanilla powder
360g stone-ground polenta (I like Biona
    Organic Polenta Bramata)
420g ground almonds
12 teaspoons ground arrowroot

FOR THE BLUEBERRY JAM

250g blueberries
1 tablespoon maple syrup
2 tablespoons chia seeds

FOR THE CARAMEL ICING

10 medjool dates, pitted
3 tablespoons almond milk
4 tablespoons cashew butter
pinch of salt

FOR THE COCONUT ICING

3 tablespoons cashew butter
250g coconut yogurt
3 tablespoons coconut sugar
½ teaspoon vanilla powder

TO DECORATE

blueberries
coconut sugar
coconut chips

Preheat the oven to 195°C (fan 175°C). Oil 3 x 20cm cake tins, or line with baking parchment. Put the chia into a mug with 8 tablespoons of water. Leave for 20 minutes until the seeds expand and form a gel. Gently melt the 4½ tablespoons of coconut oil.

In a large bowl, mix all the cake ingredients, including the chia and coconut oil. Stir until smooth. Divide between the prepared tins and bake for 35–40 minutes until golden; a knife poked in should come out clean.

Meanwhile, for the jam, heat the ingredients together in a pan for about 10 minutes until a thick sticky jam forms, then set aside to cool. For the caramel icing, put all the ingredients in a food processor. Blend until smooth. For the coconut icing, blend the ingredients together or – if your cashew butter isn't too solid – just stir them. Chill to set a bit.

When the cakes are cooked, let cool in the tins, then remove from the tins.

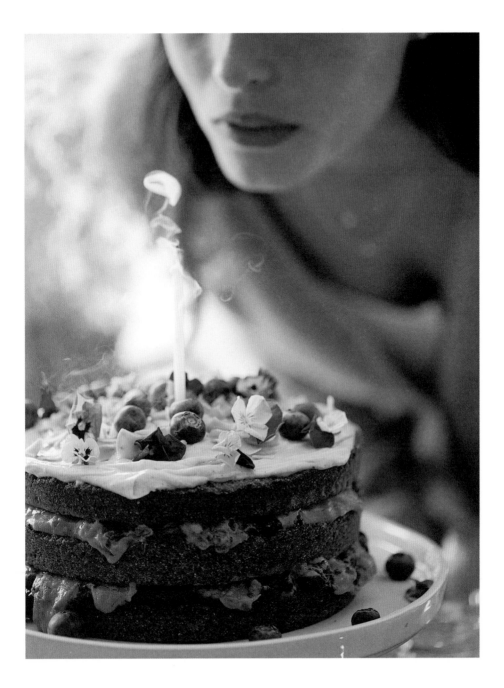

Thickly spread jam on a cake (with some caramel icing, if you like), then put another on top. Spread with caramel icing, then put the last cake on top. Spread with coconut icing. Decorate with blueberries, a sprinkling of coconut sugar and coconut chips. Enjoy!

CLEVER COOKING

Don't make the layers of the cake too thick. You want them to be 2.5cm or so deep, any more and the cake may topple, plus it will be hard to eat!

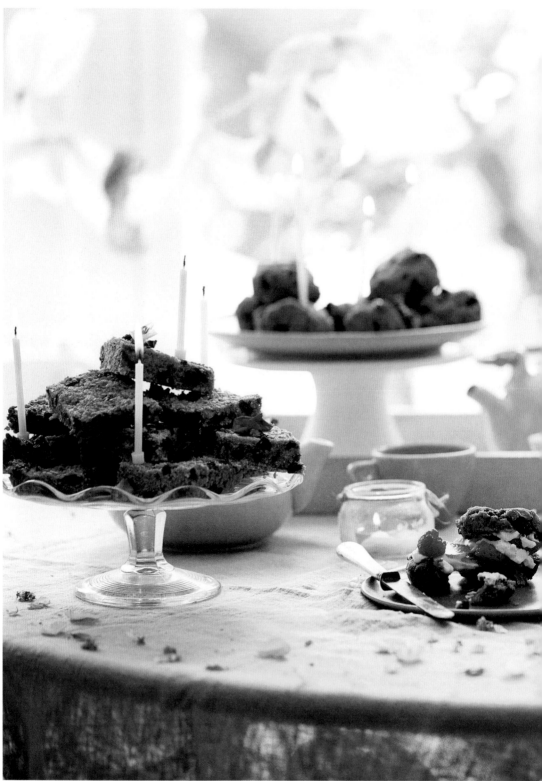

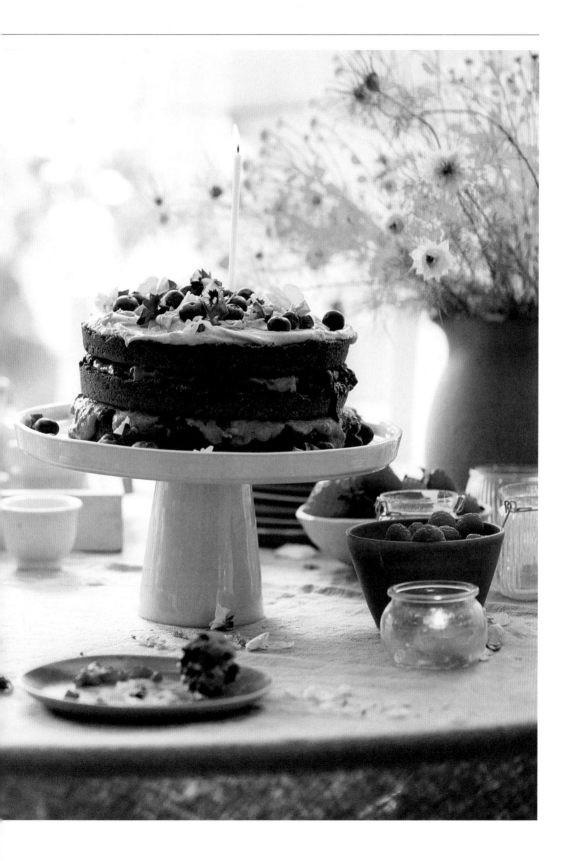

BLUEBERRY SCONES WITH VANILLA COCONUT CREAM

*Scones always feel like a pretty vital part of an afternoon tea, they're just so
quintessentially British, so I had to include them in this menu. These are delicious, but
not overly sweet, which is refreshing if you're serving them with flapjacks and cake
(pages 229 and 230)! The versatile vanilla cream works with most cakes or desserts.*

Makes 10

3 heaped tablespoons coconut oil, plus
    more for the muffin tray (optional)
300g brown rice flour
6 tablespoons coconut sugar
2 teaspoons ground arrowroot
3 teaspoons vanilla powder
2 teaspoons ground cinnamon
1 teaspoon baking powder
pinch of salt
140ml almond milk (or oat milk or other
    plant-based milk if you are nut-free)
finely grated zest of 1 unwaxed lemon,
    plus the juice of ½ lemon
3 teaspoons maple syrup
150g blueberries
80g raisins

VANILLA COCONUT CREAM
250g coconut yogurt
1 teaspoon vanilla powder
1 tablespoon pale runny honey (this looks
    nicer if it's a clearer honey)

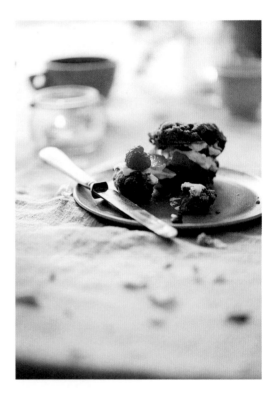

Preheat the oven to 200°C (fan 180°C). Oil a
muffin tray with coconut oil.

In a bowl, stir the dry ingredients together
(not the blueberries or raisins) so they're well
and truly mixed.

Add the solid 3 tablespoons of coconut oil
and use your hands to rub it in, lifting your
hands into the air over the bowl and rubbing
with your fingertips, until the mixture starts to
resemble breadcrumbs.

Pour in the almond milk, lemon zest and
juice and maple syrup and bring it all
together, kneading it in the bowl. Work in the
blueberries and raisins.

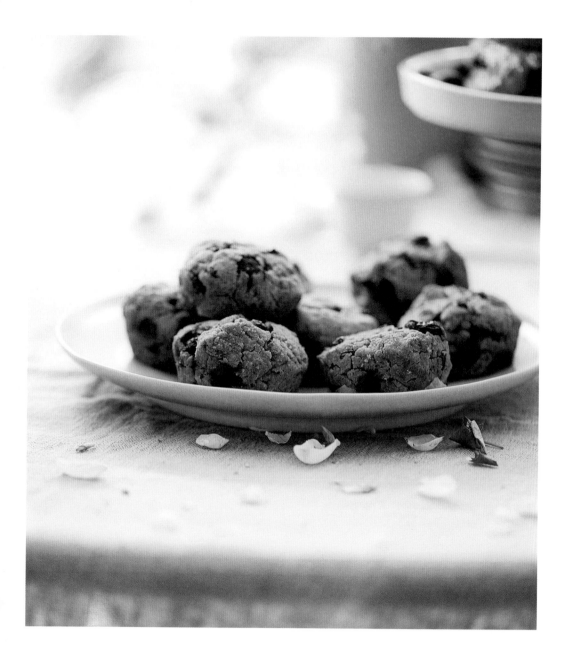

Using a dessertspoon, scoop up a generous spoonful of the mixture, and drop it into a hollow of the muffin tray, smoothing down the top of the scone with the back of a spoon. You should be able to make 10.

Pop them in the oven for 25 minutes, but check on them after 20 minutes: they should be turning golden brown when they're done. Remove from the oven and let cool.

Meanwhile, in a bowl, beat all the ingredients for the vanilla coconut cream together with a whisk. Cover and keep in the fridge until ready to use. Serve the scones with the cream, adding fresh berries, if you like.

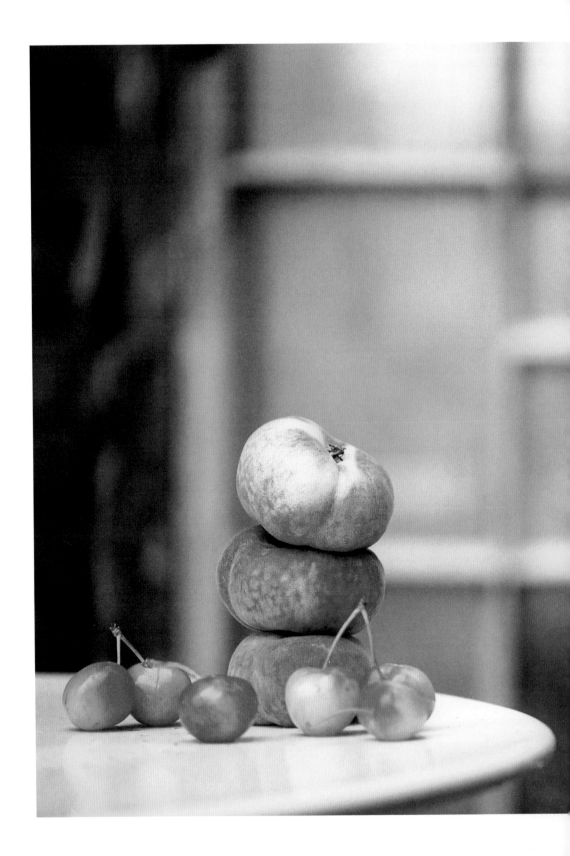

SWEETS

THE BEST WAY TO END A MEAL!

WATERMELON & MINT GRANITA

*A wonderfully light, refreshing dessert, which requires only three simple ingredients.
It's ideal for warm summer nights with friends, especially alongside a lovely cocktail
or mocktail (pages 214–219). I think it's the perfect finish to my garden party supper
of Marinated Cauliflower Steaks with Chilli Quinoa and Sun-dried Tomato & Butter
Bean Hummus (pages 134 and 137).*

Serves 4

NUT-FREE

3g fresh sprigs of mint, plus more
   to serve (optional)
about 500g watermelon
1 tbsp honey

Place the mint leaves into a measuring jug
and pour over 150ml of just-boiled water.
Give it a stir and let it steep for 10 minutes.

Meanwhile, cut the rind off the watermelon
and discard it. Slice up the flesh, making
sure you remove all the pips. Put the
watermelon chunks into a food processor
and whizz up until it's all liquid.

Remove the mint leaves from the water and
discard, then stir the honey into the water
until it dissolves. Stir the mint-infused honey
water and puréed watermelon together,
pour into a large, lidded freezable container,
put the lid on and put it in the freezer.

After 1 hour, remove from the freezer. Scrape
off any frozen bits around the sides and mix
in with the rest of the liquid, then return it to
the freezer. Keep doing this every hour until
you have lovely icy flakes, which you can
then tumble into glasses to serve. Garnish
with mint leaves, if you like.

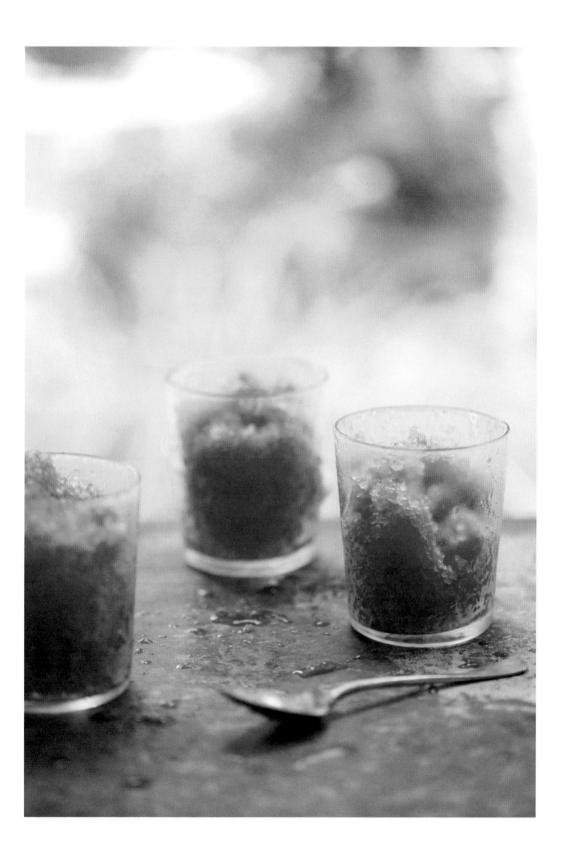

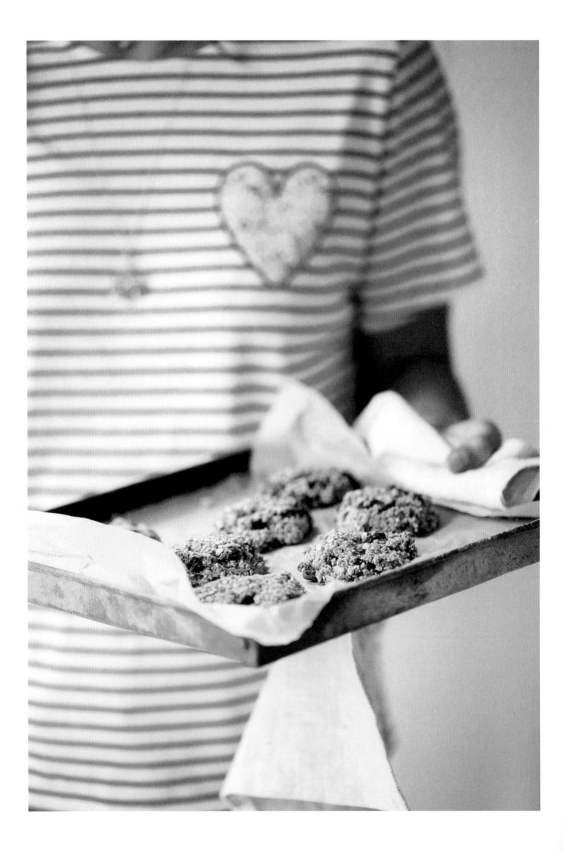

ORANGE & CARDAMOM COOKIES

These are a great staple to have in the house. They're not especially indulgent or impressive, instead they're moreish little oaty bites that sate an afternoon sweet tooth or a post-dinner snack attack. The mix of orange, lemon, cardamom and cinnamon flavours them so nicely, while the honey and raisins add a perfect sweetness.

Makes 10–12

NUT-FREE

3–5 cardamom pods, to taste (depending on how strong you want the flavour)

300g oats

6 tablespoons honey

finely grated zest of 1 unwaxed lemon, plus juice of ½ lemon

finely grated zest of 1 unwaxed orange, plus juice of ½ orange

2 tablespoon chia seeds

3 tablespoons coconut oil, melted

2 teaspoons ground cinnamon

6 tablespoons plant-based milk

40g raisins

Preheat the oven to 200°C (fan 180°C). Line a baking tray with baking parchment.

Use the flat side of a knife to crush the cardamom pods. Once each opens, take the seeds out and grind in a pestle and mortar.

Place 200g of the oats into a food processor and whizz for 30 seconds or so, until they form a flour.

Place the ground cardamom and ground oats in a large bowl and add all the remaining ingredients, not forgetting the remaining 100g of whole oats. Stir well until a nice sticky mix forms. It should be damp, rather than wet or runny.

Scoop 1 tablespoon of the mix into your hand, roll it into a ball, then place it on the prepared tray and flatten it down. Repeat to make 10–12 cookies.

Bake for 20–25 minutes. Leave on the tray until cold, so they firm up, then serve.

CLEVER COOKING

Always zest unwaxed citrus fruit before juicing it; as once you've taken the juice out it's almost impossible to zest the fruit shells.

MIX IT UP

Try smothering the cookies with a thick layer of almond butter and eating them as an afternoon snack… it's amazing!

PAN-FRIED CARDAMOM & HONEY APPLES

A lovely warming pudding, ideal if you want something sweet to end your meal but don't fancy spending ages chopping and prepping; or if you're keen to finish with something light. I love this served with coconut yogurt, a sprinkling of toasted nuts and sunflower seeds and a little drizzle of honey. Try making extra, so you can enjoy the leftovers as a treat with your porridge the next morning!

Serves 4

NUT-FREE

1 tablespoon coconut oil

1½ teaspoons ground cardamom

1½ teaspoons ground cinnamon

2 tablespoons honey

4 apples, cored and sliced into chucks

Melt the coconut oil in a large frying pan, then add the spices and honey and stir to mix. Drop in the apple chunks.

Cook everything for about 10 minutes, until the apples are soft. Serve with coconut yogurt and toasted seeds or nuts, if you like.

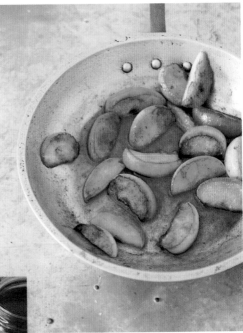

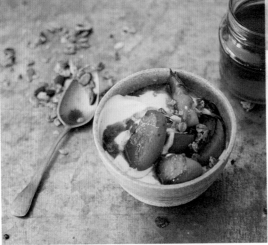

CLEVER COOKING

For this recipe, make sure you use pre-ground cardamom rather than the seeds of cardamom pods, as you need a super-fine texture. (You can grind your own seeds, but you'll have to make sure they're properly ground into a powder, then sifted, rather than just being roughly crushed.)

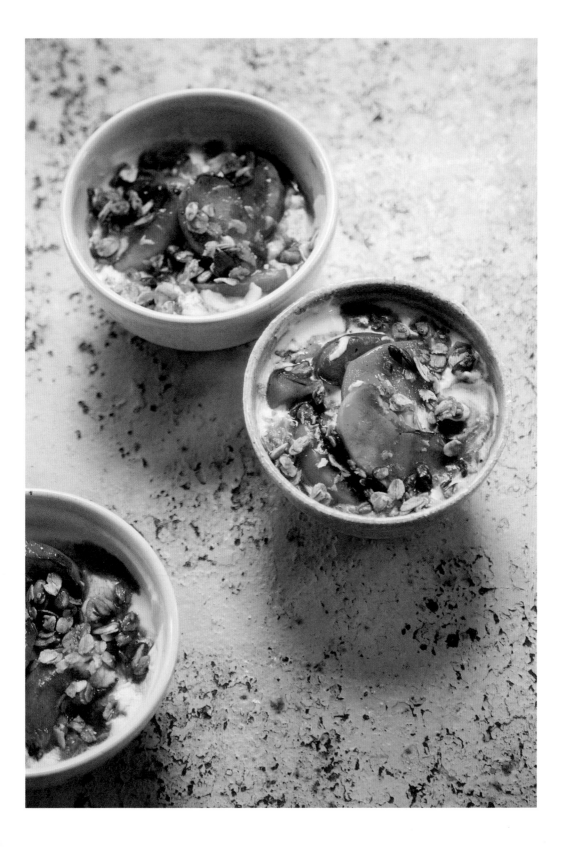

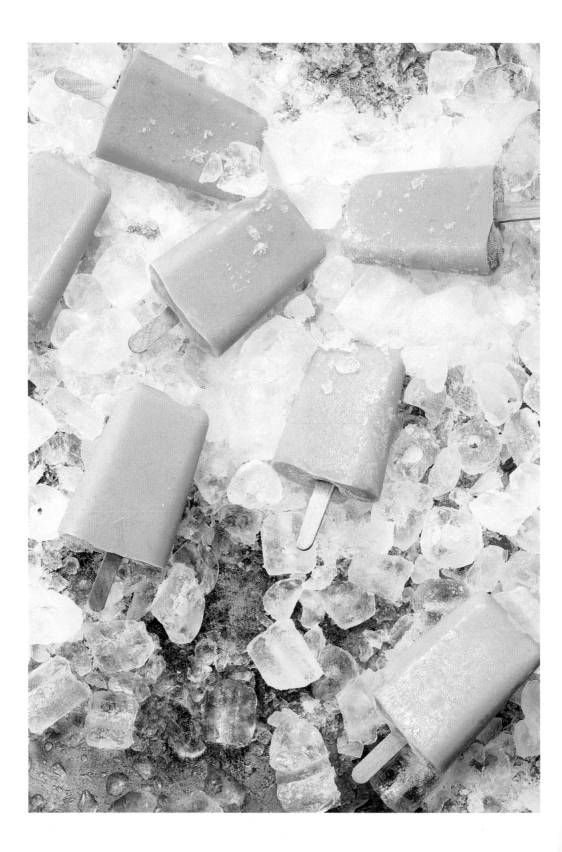

COCONUT & MANGO ICE LOLLIES

These are a summer staple. They're unbelievably simple to make, all you need to do is blend four ingredients together and then leave them to freeze solid until you're ready to enjoy. I love knowing I have a little stash of these in the freezer, too, so that as soon as the weather heats up I can cool off with one of them. They make a great end to a curry.

Makes 6

NUT-FREE

1 ripe banana (about 200g)
1 ripe mango (about 320g)
200ml coconut milk
1 tablespoon honey

Simply peel the banana, and peel and pit the mango, and roughly chop both.

Place all the ingredients into a blender and blend for 1 minute until smooth.

Pour into ice-lolly moulds and freeze for about 5 hours to set.

SUPER SPEEDY
10 minutes, plus freezing

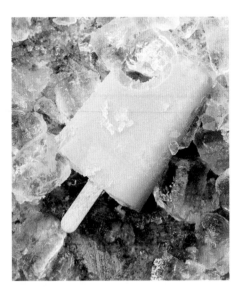

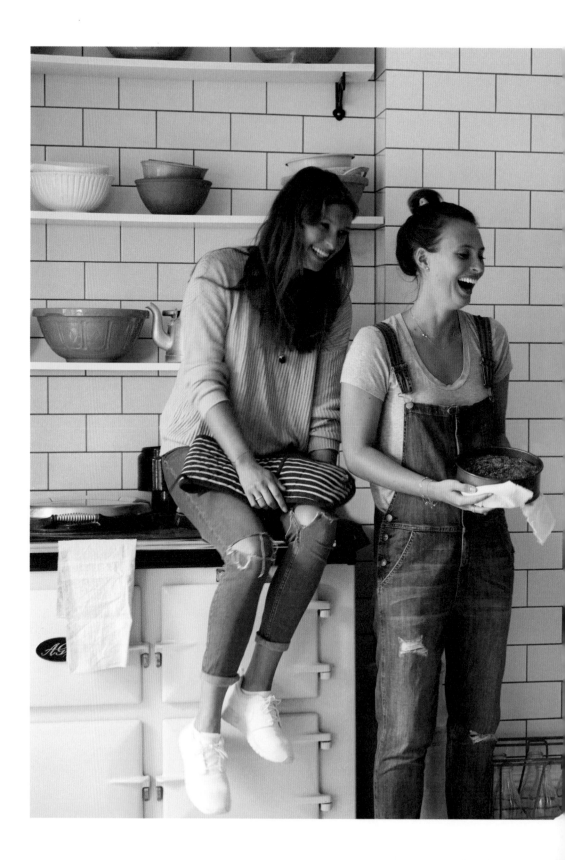

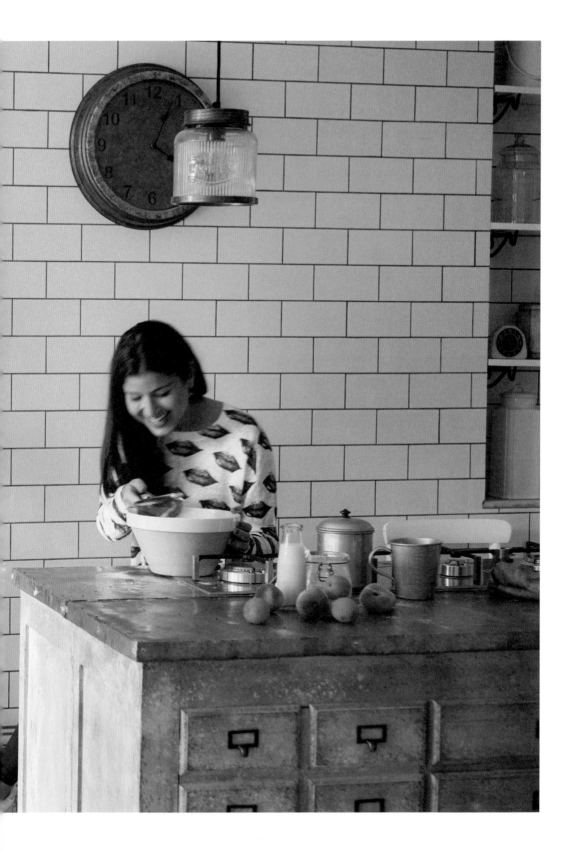

SALTED MACA & TAHINI FUDGE

Definitely one of my favourite recipes in this book, this is completely delicious and utterly addictive. The first time I made this fudge I couldn't stop thinking about it for weeks afterwards, I would literally dream of it, so I had to keep making it time and again to sate my cravings! This is a great treat option if you just want a little sweet bite, rather than a big dessert, or eat it with tea and coffee afterwards if you want both!

Makes 16–20 pieces

200g cashew nuts
1½ teaspoons vanilla powder
6 medjool dates, pitted
2 tablespoons maca powder
3 tablespoons coconut sugar
3 tablespoons tahini
sea salt flakes

Preheat the oven to 220°C (fan 200°C). Line a lunch box or loaf tin with cling film.

Spread the cashews on a baking tray and cook at the top of the oven for 5 minutes, or until they start to turn golden brown. Remove from the oven and leave to cool. Place them in a powerful food processor with the vanilla powder and blend until they form a creamy cashew butter.

Add the dates, maca, coconut sugar and tahini to the food processor and blend for another 5 minutes until the dates have broken down and the mixture is smooth (it may be a bit crumbly but that's OK!).

Spoon the mixture into the prepared box or tin, pressing it down with a spatula to make it even. Sprinkle the top with sea salt flakes and place in the freezer for 2 hours to firm up.

Store the fudge in the freezer, taking it out 30 minutes prior to serving to soften a little bit before eating. Enjoy!

CLEVER COOKING

These look super-cute and are easier to take with you out and about if you wrap them individually in twists of baking parchment.

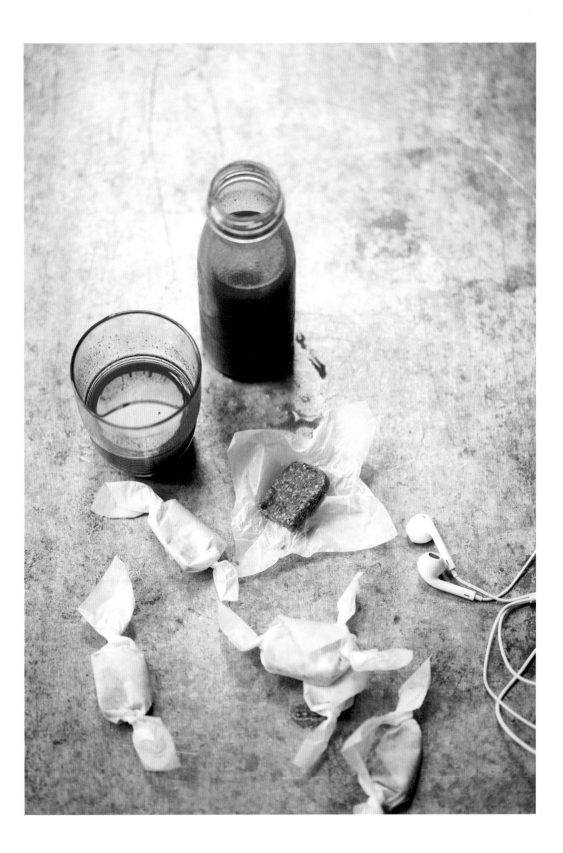

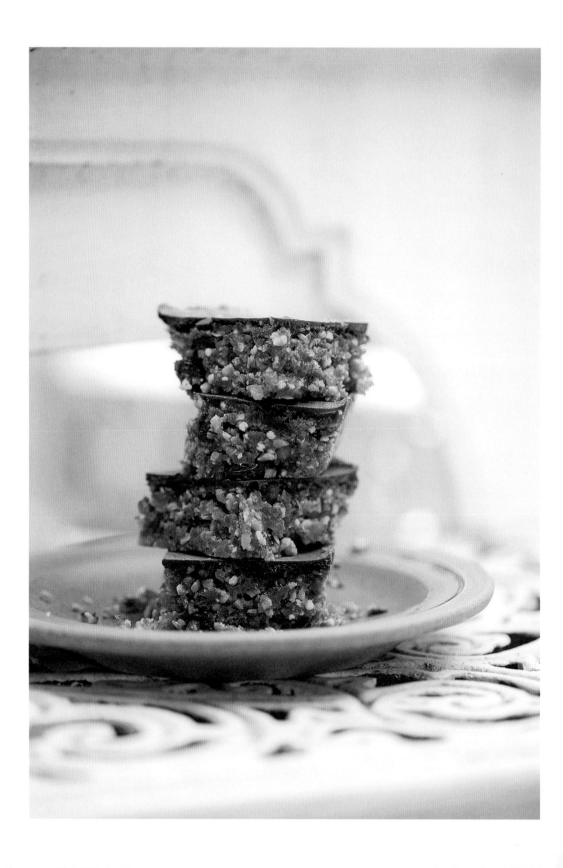

QUINOA, HAZELNUT & CACAO BARS

Another favourite from this book. These slip down too easily, which can be a little dangerous, and half of them can end up disappearing before you've even shared them around! The bottom layer is amazing: nicely sweet but not sickly and there's such a wonderful array of flavours and textures (I especially love the chewy bites of dried apricots). The chocolate on top adds an indulgent touch, finishing the bars off perfectly.

Makes 20

FOR THE BASE

160g hazelnuts

12 medjool dates, pitted

4 tablespoons almond butter

2 tablespoons tahini

5 tablespoons coconut oil

40g puffed quinoa

50g sesame seeds

60g raisins

150g dried apricots (preferably unsulphured), finely chopped

FOR THE CHOCOLATE LAYER

200g cacao butter

5 tablespoons raw cacao powder

6 tablespoons maple syrup

pinch of salt

Preheat the oven to 200°C (fan 180°C). Line a regular-sized 30 x 20cm baking tray with baking parchment.

Roast the hazelnuts on another baking tray for 10 minutes, then remove from the oven and leave to cool.

Tip the hazelnuts into a food processor and pulse until broken down into chunks. Put into a large mixing bowl.

Now put the dates into the food processor with the almond butter, tahini and coconut oil. Blend for a minute or so until a smooth paste forms, then add to the hazelnuts in the large mixing bowl. Add all the other base ingredients to the bowl and mix together until completely combined.

Press the mixture into the prepared tray, making sure it is even and quite firmly packed. Place in the fridge to set.

Meanwhile, make the chocolate layer. Simply place the cacao butter, cacao powder, maple syrup and salt into a saucepan and place over a really gentle heat until they have melted together; don't let them come to the boil. Remove the base layer from the fridge and pour the chocolate over the top, then return to the fridge for another 1½ hours to let the chocolate layer set.

Cut into 20 bars to serve. Store any leftovers in the fridge.

PISTACHIO & ORANGE TRUFFLE BITES

The best post-dinner treat to serve with tea and coffee. They're gooey and indulgent with an ever-so-slightly chewy texture inside and a crunchy outside. They have smooth chocolatey centres and are rolled in crumbled pistachios to give the perfect finish.

Makes 16–18

50g pistachio nuts
12 medjool dates, pitted and chopped
finely grated zest of 1 unwaxed orange,
    plus juice of ½ orange
1 teaspoon coconut oil
3 tablespoons raw cacao powder

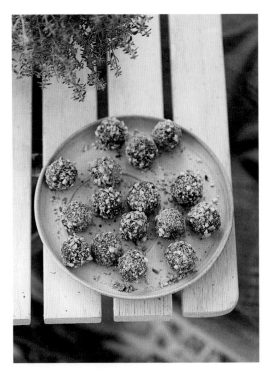

Put the nuts in a food processor and whizz to a crumb-like consistency. Don't worry if they're not all the same size; they're for the truffle coating, so different-sized crumbs will add character! When you're happy with the size, tip them into a bowl and set aside.

Throw the dates, orange zest, coconut oil and cacao powder into the processor and whizz it all together. If it gets stuck, use a spatula to push it down towards the blades again and give it another whizz. When it's starting to stick together, squeeze in the orange juice and whizz again until it's a nice sticky consistency that you can roll into balls.

Get a baking sheet ready and wet your hands slightly so that the mixture is easy to roll into balls. Use a teaspoon to get a nice amount together and roll it into a ball. Drop into the nut crumbs and roll it around to coat. Set it on the baking sheet. Repeat to use all the mix.

Place the baking sheet in the fridge to chill for at least 30 minutes before serving.

MIX IT UP
You can use any nuts you have to hand if you don't want to buy pistachios, but the colour of the pistachios makes these look fancy! Or use a mix of chopped pistachios and cashews with pistachio nibs if you want to go all out with eye-catchingly different textures.

SUPER SPEEDY
15 minutes, plus chilling time

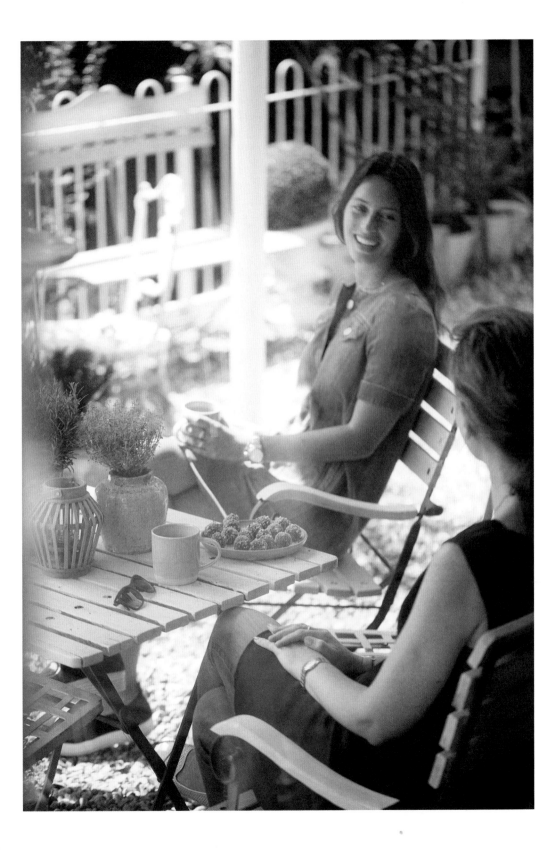

BERRIES WITH CREAMY CHOCOLATE SAUCE & TOASTED NUTS

The perfect dessert for a weekday supper with friends. It just takes fifteen minutes or so to prepare, plus it can't really go wrong, which is a nice feeling when you're a bit tight on time and tired after a long day at work! I like serving this in little bowls, with a bright layer of fresh berries on the bottom and a generous drizzling of warm chocolate sauce and crushed nuts on top. There's nothing fancy about it, but it hits the spot every time.

Serves 4

50g pecans
50g almonds
3 tablespoons coconut oil
50g raw cacao powder
6 tablespoons maple syrup
1 tablespoon almond butter, or any other
nut butter
50ml plant-based milk (I used almond milk)
400g berries (I used blueberries and
raspberries, but any fruit works)

Preheat the oven to 200°C (fan 180°C).

Place the pecans and almonds on a baking tray and bake for about 10 minutes, until crunchy. Set aside to cool.

Now put the coconut oil, cacao powder, maple syrup and almond butter into a saucepan and place over a gentle heat for a few minutes until it has all melted. Then take off the heat and whisk in the almond milk to make a smooth sauce.

Roughly chop the nuts, then assemble the dessert. Tumble the berries into 4 bowls, pour over the chocolate sauce, then sprinkle with the chopped nuts. What a treat!

PAN TO PLATE
15 minutes

CLEVER COOKING
This is a great way to use up any leftovers in the house. All fruit works perfectly in this recipe, from grapes to blackberries, strawberries... or indeed anything else you have in the fridge!

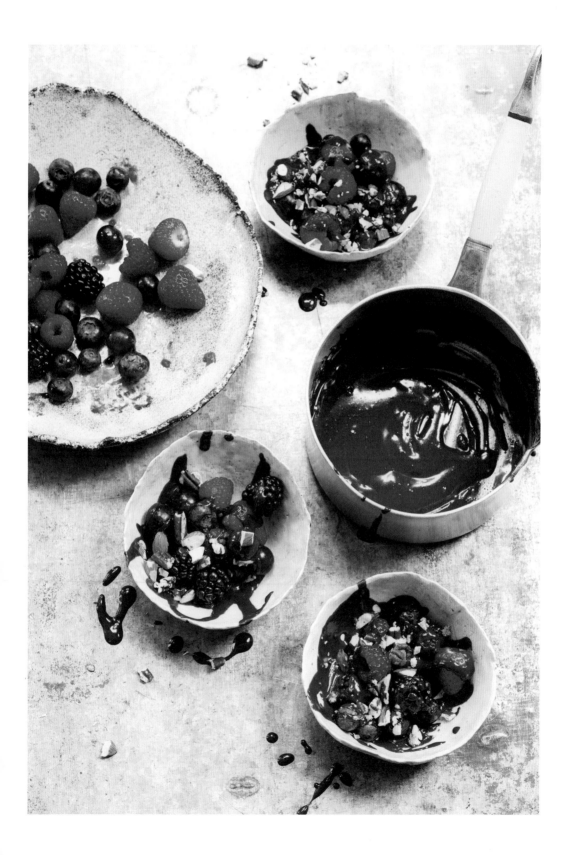

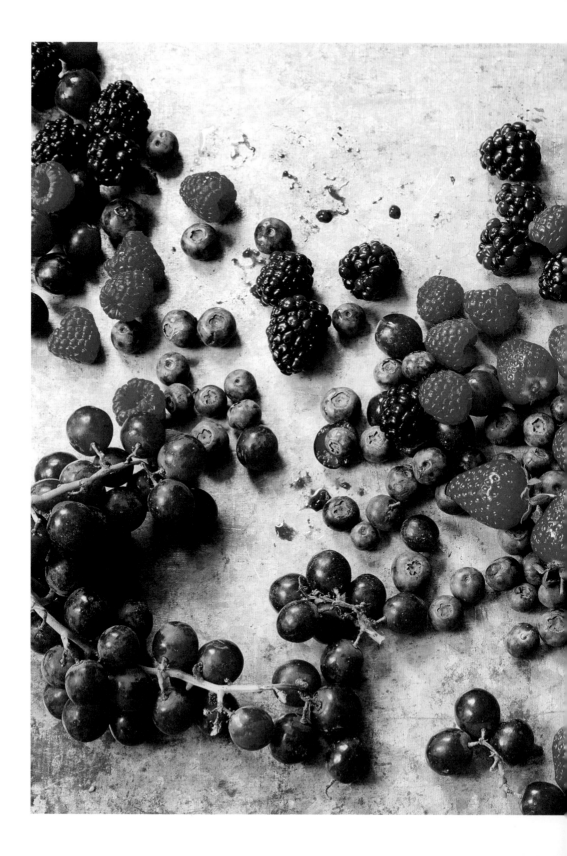

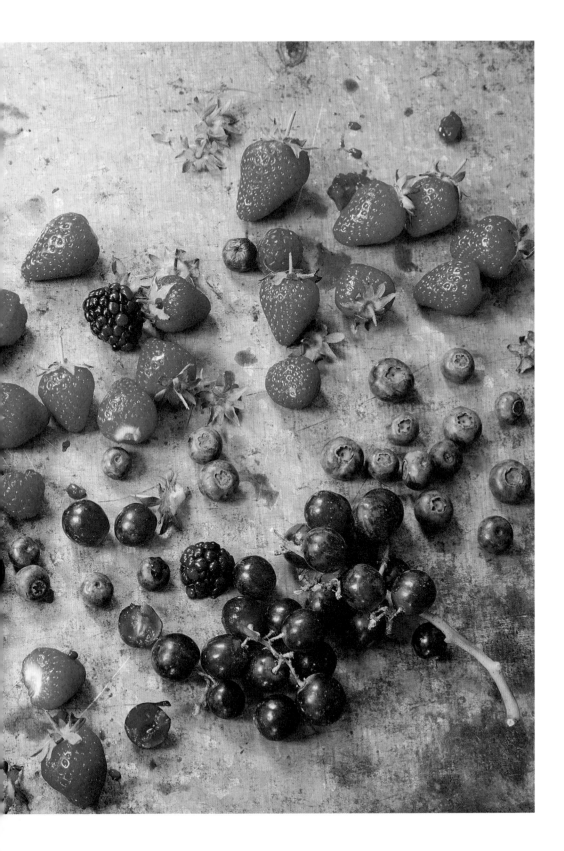

PEACH & COCONUT TART

This is utter heaven. It's just made to share with friends on a warm summer's day, so you can sit outside and enjoy every bite. It's also a great recipe for those of you who don't like overly sweet desserts, but it's still bursting with flavour. I love serving this slightly warm, with generous scoops of coconut ice cream.

Makes 1 large tart / Serves 12

6 peaches
7 tablespoons coconut oil
4 tablespoons maple syrup
sprinkle of ground cinnamon
2 tablespoons chia seeds
100g buckwheat flour
200g ground almonds
3 teaspoons vanilla powder
4 tablespoons coconut sugar
75g desiccated coconut
10g coconut chips

Preheat the oven to 200°C (fan 180°C). Have a 26 x 28cm ovenproof baking dish to hand.

Halve and pit the peaches, then slice them. Heat 1 tablespoon of the coconut oil and 1 tablespoon of the maple syrup in a pan and add the peach slices and cinnamon. Cook for 10 minutes, until the fruit begins to soften but still holds its shape.

In a small bowl, mix the chia seeds with 6 tablespoons of water. Leave for 20 minutes until the seeds expand and form a gel.

Pour the flour, ground almonds, vanilla, coconut sugar and remaining 6 tablespoons of coconut oil and 3 tablespoons of maple syrup into a food processor and blitz until everything has mixed together.

Remove 85g of the mix, stir it with the desiccated coconut in a bowl and set aside.

Once the chia seeds have soaked up the water, add this to the remaining mixture in the food processor and mix again.

Cut out a sheet of baking parchment to fit the baking dish. Remove the mixture from the food processor and roll it out on to the baking parchment with a rolling pin, until 2.5cm thick and wide enough to fit the baking dish.

Place the rolled-out mixture on its baking parchment base into the dish, then bake for 10 minutes. Remove from the oven and leave to cool for 5 minutes before scattering half the cooked peaches over the top, squashing down slightly with the back of a wooden spoon. Sprinkle the desiccated coconut mixture on top and bake for 20 minutes.

Remove from the oven, add the other half of the peaches, sprinkle with the coconut chips and bake for a final 12 minutes.

Remove from the oven and leave to cool for about 20 minutes. Then slice, serve and enjoy. Store in an airtight container in the fridge to avoid it going soft.

MIX IT UP
Try serving the Melting Middle sauce from the Sticky Toffee Pudding with this (page 270); they taste incredible together!

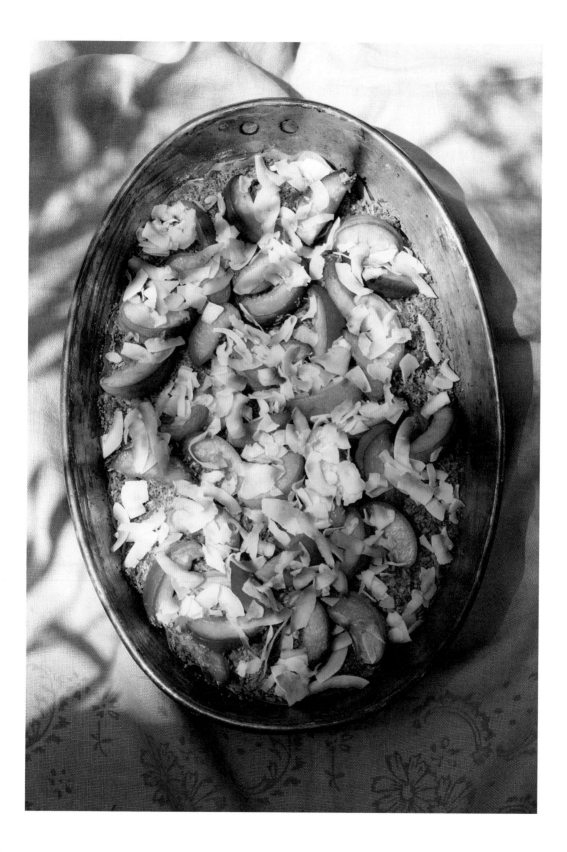

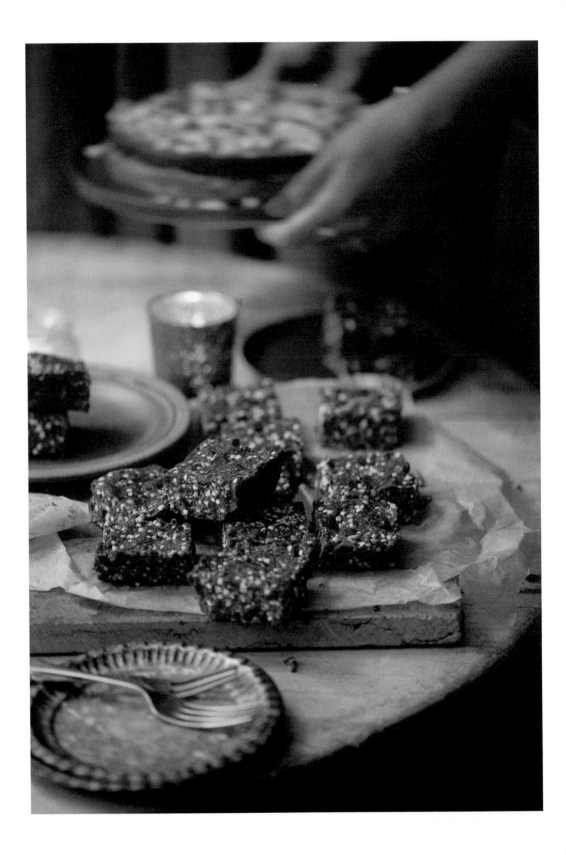

ALMOND BUTTER ROCKY ROADS

It's hard to describe how much I love these. I could happily eat an entire tray in one sitting… and have done too many times! Each square is wonderfully gooey and chocolatey, with sweet raisins and crunchy toasted buckwheat bites adding extra texture and substance. All I can say is that you just have to go and make them; I promise you'll adore them, too. You can also make them nut-free, with just a couple of tweaks.

Makes 15

150g buckwheat groats

100g cacao butter

200g oats

100g pecans (or pumpkin seeds, if you're nut-free)

300g medjool dates, pitted

2 heaped tablespoons almond butter (or tahini, if you're nut-free)

5 tablespoons maple syrup

5 tablespoons raw cacao powder

pinch of sea salt

100g raisins

Preheat the oven to 200°C (fan 180°C). Pour the buckwheat groats evenly on to a baking tray and bake for 10 minutes, giving the tray a shake halfway through so they all get a bit of colour.

Meanwhile, place the cacao butter in a saucepan and heat gently until melted.

Pour the oats and pecans into a food processor and blitz until they're fully ground down. Add the dates, almond butter, maple syrup, cacao powder, melted cacao butter and salt. Blitz together to form a really smooth and sticky consistency.

Pour the mixture into a large bowl with the raisins and toasted buckwheat and mix well.

Line a 20cm square brownie tin with baking parchment, pour in the mixture and smooth it down with a spatula. The mix can be pretty sticky, so make sure you press it well into all the corners. Freeze for about 1 hour, then slice into 15 pieces to serve.

PB & J CAKE

*So chocolatey and delicious. Using a mix of dates, banana, peanut butter and coconut oil
makes the sponge really gooey and fudgy, which is amazing… though it's pretty rich.
The icing is pretty special, too. I use two layers of goodness to ice it: one mix of peanut
butter, maple and vanilla icing and another of smashed raspberries with coconut sugar;
you can only image how good they taste together, especially with the rich chocolate
sponge. It's the perfect treat for any celebratory meal, or your reward after
a weekend baking session.*

Makes 1 cake

FOR THE CAKE

1 tablespoon coconut oil, plus more
   for the tins
150g oats
150g ground almonds
200ml brown rice milk
2 ripe avocados, peeled and pitted

10 medjool dates, pitted
10 tablespoons raw cacao powder
8 tablespoons maple syrup
5 tablespoons coconut sugar
5 tablespoons peanut butter
4 tablespoons chia seeds
1 small, over-ripe banana (80g with skin on),
   peeled and mashed
pinch of salt

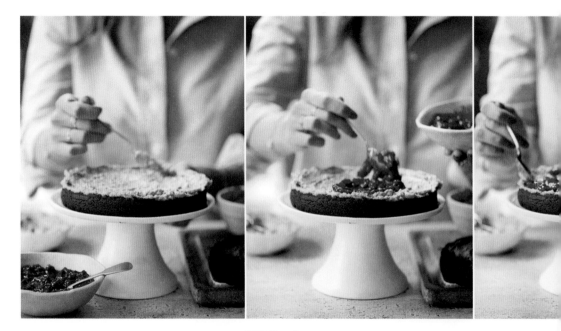

FOR THE ICING

100g cashews (soaked for 2–4 hours)
3 tablespoons maple syrup
1 teaspoon vanilla powder
½ tablespoon coconut oil
½ tablespoon coconut sugar
3 tablespoons peanut butter

FOR THE RASPBERRY LAYER

250g raspberries, plus more to serve
2 tablespoons coconut sugar,
   plus more to serve

Preheat the oven to 200°C (fan 180°C). Oil 2 x 20–22cm cake tins with coconut oil.

Tip the oats into a food processor and blend until a flour forms. Add all the other ingredients – not forgetting the 1 tablespoon of coconut oil – and blend until a thick, chocolatey mix forms. Fill each of the prepared tins with half the batter.

Place the cakes in the oven and bake for about 50 minutes; a knife poked in should come out clean. Let the cakes cool in the tins, they'll finish setting while they cool.

Meanwhile, make the icing. Drain the cashews and tip into a blender. Add all the other ingredients with 60ml of water. Blitz, then scrape out into a bowl and let it sit in the fridge for 10 minutes or so to firm up.

For the raspberry layer, mash the raspberries on a plate, stirring in the coconut sugar.

Finally, spread half the icing over the flat side of the least attractive cake, then spread half the mashed raspberries over it. Place the other cake on top, flat bases together, and do the same again. Arrange some raspberries over the top. I like to sprinkle a little extra coconut sugar on top as a final flourish, as it looks beautiful.

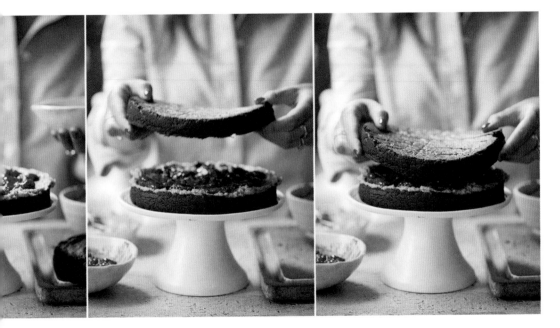

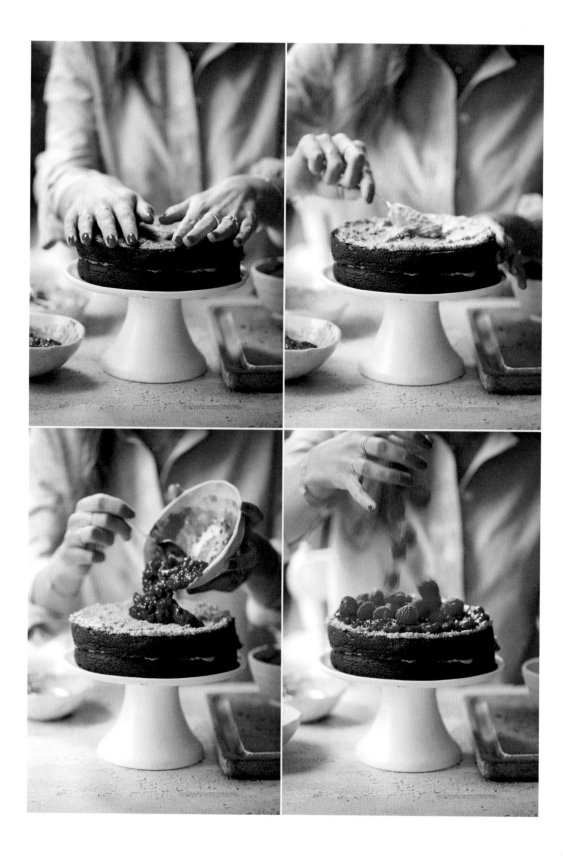

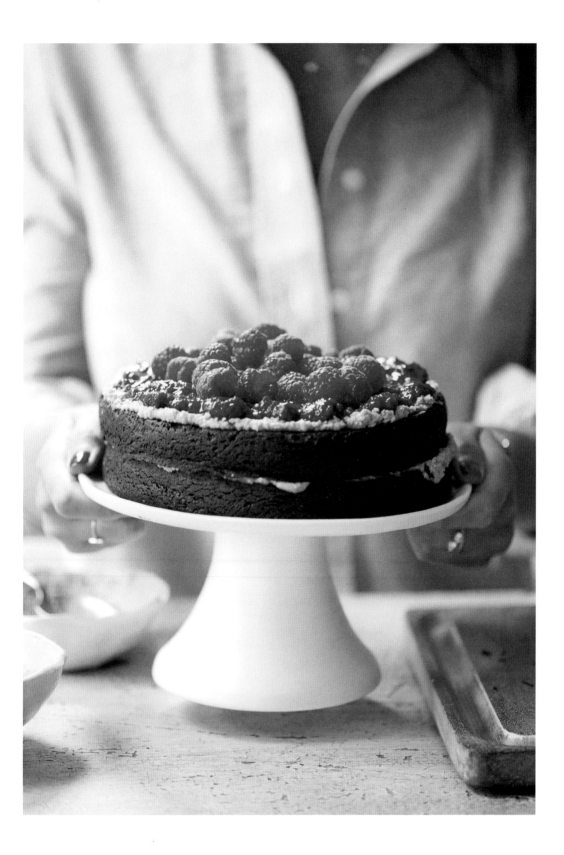

CHOCOLATE ORANGE TART

Anything chocolate orange-focused is always such a winner; it's a classic combination of flavours that everyone seems to love; this creamy tart is no exception. The almond and orange base has subtle hints of cacao, coconut and maple, which perfectly complement the sweet, creamy middle. The tart is then finished off with a beautiful scattering of orange zest and salt, which heighten the flavours and make it look perfect.

Serves 10–12

FOR THE BASE

2 tablespoons coconut oil, plus more
   for the tin
150g almonds
2 tablespoons raw cacao powder
150g medjool dates, pitted
finely grated zest of 1 unwaxed orange,
   plus juice of ½ orange
pinch of salt
1 tablespoon maple syrup

FOR THE MIDDLE LAYER

2 ripe avocados
2 tablespoons coconut oil
4 tablespoons date syrup
2 tablespoons honey
4 heaped tablespoons raw cacao powder
finely grated zest and juice of
   2 unwaxed oranges
pinch of salt
2 tablespoons peanut or almond butter

TO DECORATE

finely grated zest of ½ unwaxed orange
pinch of sea salt flakes

Oil a 20cm springform cake tin with coconut oil, or line it with baking parchment.

Make the base. Start by blitzing the almonds in a food processor until they form a chunky flour, then add all the other ingredients – not forgetting the 2 tablespoons of coconut oil – and blend until a sticky mix forms. Use a spatula to firmly press the mix down into the prepared tin. Place in the freezer for 30 minutes to allow the tart base to set.

Meanwhile, make the middle layer. Pit and peel the avocados, then place them with all the other ingredients into a food processer. Blend until a smooth, creamy, mousse-like mixture forms. Pour it over the base, then return to the freezer for 1 hour to set. Take it out about 15 minutes before serving.

Grate the orange zest over the top and sprinkle with a few sea salt flakes.

Store any leftovers in the freezer.

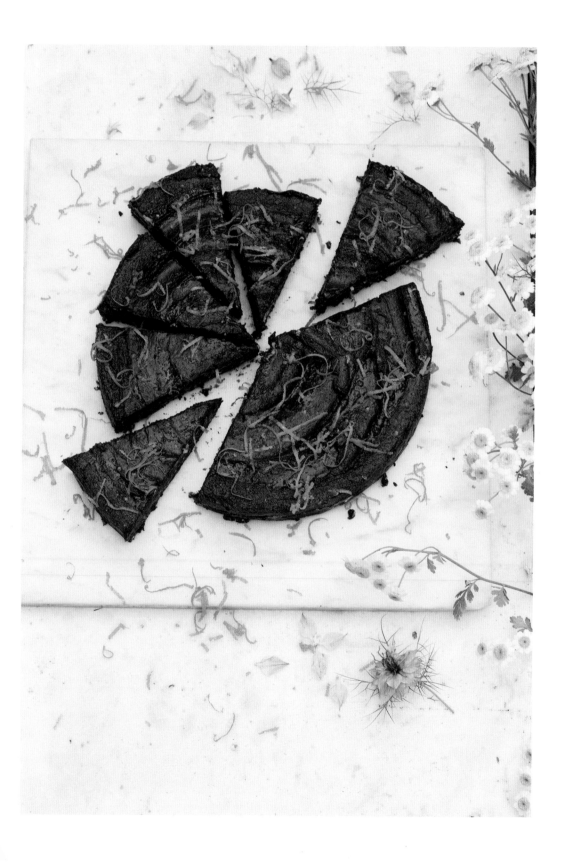

CHOCOLATE PEANUT BUTTER PIE

Who doesn't love the sound of this?! It is real indulgence: sweet, rich, nutty and
oh-so-delicious. It's also pretty filling, so you may want to cut your guests relatively small
slices to start with and serve it alongside some dollops of coconut yogurt to lighten it up.
My ultimate treat. I hope it will be yours, too!

Serves 12

FOR THE CHOCOLATE LAYER
120g coconut oil, plus more for the tin
100g raw cacao powder
30g cacao butter
1 teaspoon vanilla powder
60g peanut butter
60g honey
60g coconut sugar
pinch of salt

FOR THE BASE
200g oats
40g coconut oil
30g peanut butter
30g honey
1 teaspoon vanilla powder
pinch of salt

FOR THE MIDDLE LAYER AND TOPPING
150g peanut butter
1–2 tablespoons raw unsalted peanuts,
   roughly chopped

Oil a 20cm springform cake tin with coconut
oil, or line it with baking parchment.

Make the chocolate layer first. Simply place
all the ingredients into a saucepan over a low
heat and gently stir until melted and mixed
together. Set aside to cool and thicken.

Meanwhile, make the base. Whizz the oats
in a food processor to a flour, then add all the
other ingredients, with 2 tablespoons of water
and 2 tablespoons of the chocolate layer mix.
Blend until a sticky mix forms. Press over the
prepared tin, so it's tightly packed, then place
in the freezer for 10–15 minutes to firm up.

Spread the 150g of peanut butter evenly over
the base, then freeze for 10 minutes to set.

Finally, pour the chocolate layer over and
sprinkle with the peanuts. Let it set in the
fridge for 30 minutes before serving. Be
patient! It really does need the setting time.

Store any leftovers in the fridge or freezer.

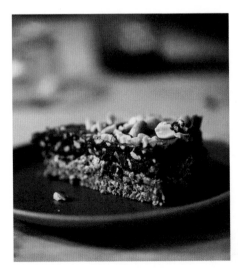

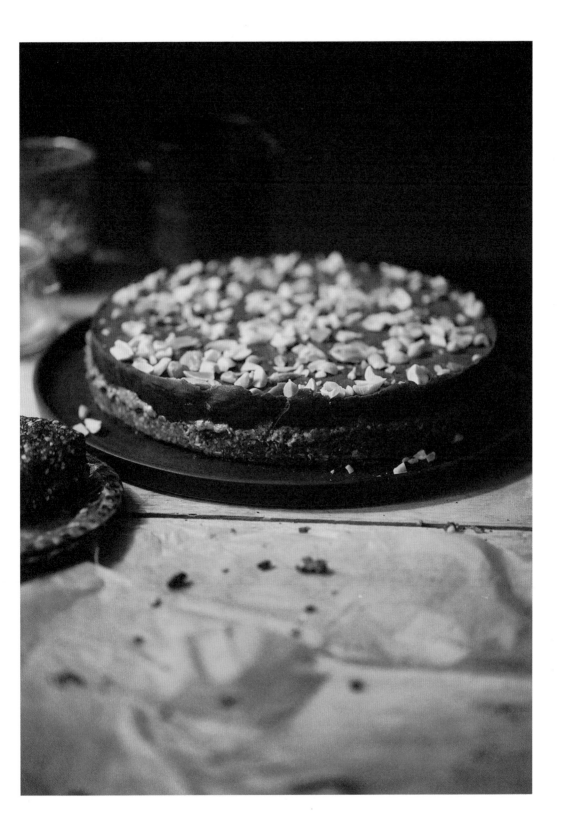

STICKY TOFFEE PUDDING

Growing up, sticky toffee pudding was mine and my siblings' favourite dessert. We were all obsessed with it and would ask for it all the time... we even used to have it on Christmas Day. I'm sure part of the reason I love it so much is that it's a celebration of sweet, sticky dates and — as lots of you know — I adore dates, so any dessert where they're the focus is always a winner in my book! This is a really indulgent way to end a meal, and absolutely nothing about it looks or tastes healthy, so it's ideal if you've got a few sceptical friends coming over and you need a real treat to serve them. It is great served with coconut yogurt or coconut ice cream, which add a lovely refreshing touch.

Serves 8

FOR THE MELTING MIDDLE SAUCE
200g medjool dates, pitted
3 tablespoons coconut oil
2 tablespoons maple syrup
2 tablespoons coconut sugar
pinch of salt

FOR THE PUDDING
200g medjool dates, pitted
2 tablespoons flax seeds
130g ground almonds
70g polenta
2 tablespoons coconut sugar
2 tablespoons maple syrup
2 tablespoons date syrup
1 teaspoon vanilla powder
pinch of salt

Start with the sauce. Place the dates in a pan with the coconut oil. Allow them to melt and warm together for about 5 minutes, until the dates are nice and soft. Pour this into a blender with the maple syrup, coconut sugar and salt, then pour in 250ml of water. Blend until a deliciously smooth, thick sauce forms.

For the pudding, put the dates in a saucepan with 250ml of water. Place over a low heat until a sticky paste forms, then set aside. In a bowl, soak the flax seeds with 4 tablespoons of water for 10 minutes, so it starts to thicken. Mix the date paste and flax seeds with all the other ingredients in a large mixing bowl.

Line a 1-litre pudding bowl with baking parchment. Spoon 5 tablespoons of the sauce into the bowl, then spoon the pudding mix on top. Tie baking parchment over the bowl with string to secure. Put it in a wide pan and fill the pan with boiling water to come halfway up the bowl. Cover, place over a medium heat and bring to a simmer. Simmer for 1½ hours. Ensure the water doesn't evaporate as it might burn the pudding or crack the bowl; check on it every 30 minutes.

Place a serving plate on top of the bowl and flip to remove the pudding. Leave it there for about 10 minutes while you reheat the sauce for drizzling over the top!

CLEVER COOKING
I often make extra sauce, as I can never get enough of it with this pudding!

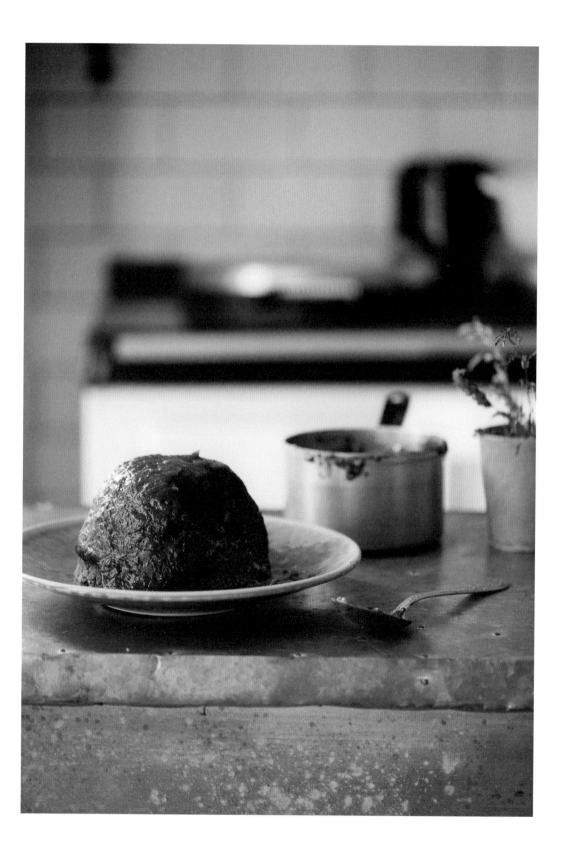

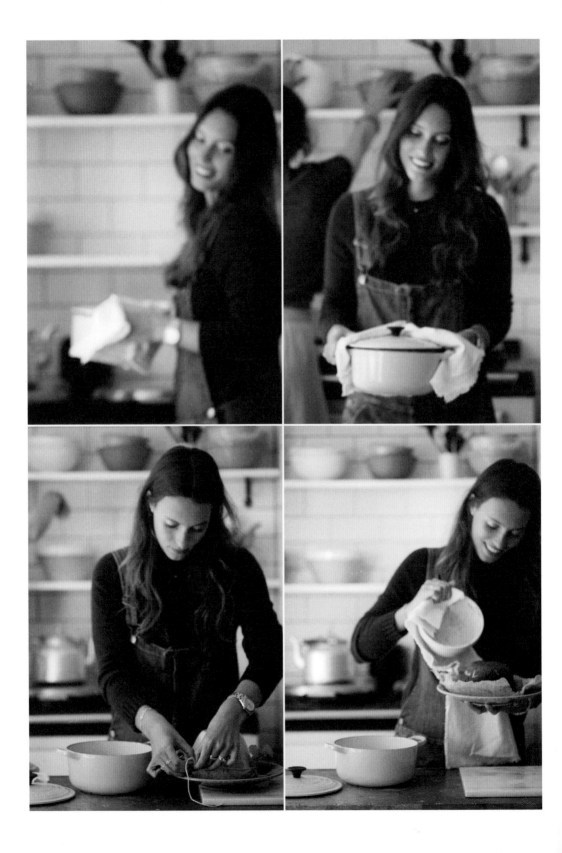

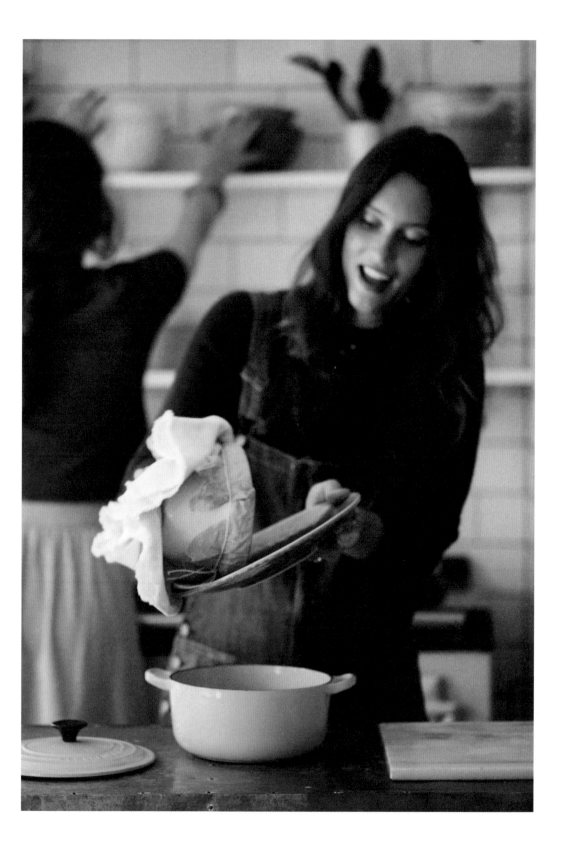

ORANGE & POLENTA CAKE

Definitely the Deliciously Ella office's favourite cake. Every time this has been made it seems to get devoured within minutes and we can't wait for it to be recipe tested again! It's lighter than the PB & J cake (page 262), with lovely hints of almond and orange. My favourite part is the orange and coconut sugar glaze, which is not only incredibly flavoursome, but also very beautiful. This works perfectly served at room temperature, but it's also amazing served straight out of the oven with some coconut or cashew ice cream for a warming treat in the winter, or even on a cool summer evening.

Serves 12

FOR THE CAKE

3 tablespoons coconut oil, plus more
 for the tin (optional)
2½ tablespoons chia seeds
1½ teaspoons apple cider vinegar
180ml almond milk
180ml maple syrup
2 teaspoons vanilla powder
270g fine polenta
300g ground almonds
7 teaspoons ground arrowroot
finely grated zest of ½ unwaxed lemon
finely grated zest and juice of
 1 unwaxed orange
pinch of salt

FOR THE GLAZE

finely grated zest and juice of
 2 unwaxed oranges
finely grated zest of 1 unwaxed lemon
4 tablespoons coconut sugar

Preheat the oven to 195°C (fan 175°C). Oil a 20cm cake tin with coconut oil, or line it with baking parchment.

Spoon the chia seeds into a cup, pour in 6 tablespoons of water and set aside for 20 minutes, until a gel forms.

Gently heat the 3 tablespoons of coconut oil until it melts.

In a large mixing bowl, combine all the cake ingredients, including the chia mixture and coconut oil. Stir until combined and smooth.

Spoon into the prepared tin and bake for 45–50 minutes until golden brown and a knife poked into the middle comes out clean.

Meanwhile, make the glaze. Gently heat the orange zest and juice, lemon zest and coconut sugar in a saucepan until the sugar dissolves and a thin syrup forms.

When the cake is cooked, remove it from the oven and let it cool for 20 minutes in the tin on a cooling rack, before evenly drizzling over the syrup and zest, removing from the tin and serving.

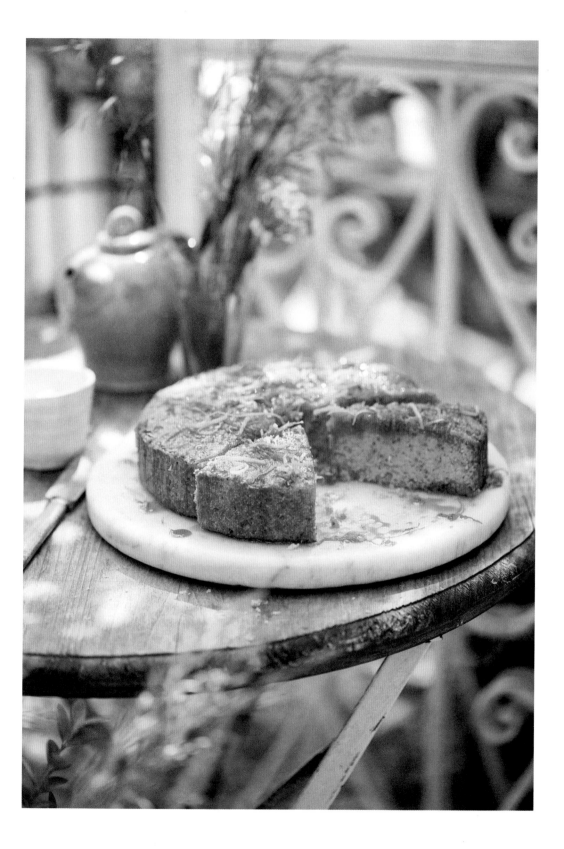

ICE CREAM SUNDAES

This is a pretty exciting dessert, filled with chewy bites of hazelnut brownie, soft scoops of banana ice cream infused with chunks of dates and your favourite nut butter, creamy chocolate sauce and then a sprinkling of toasted hazelnuts, coconut chips and a handful of sweet berries. YUM! It's a little fussy to make as there are a few different elements to it, but it's so worth doing every now and again when you want something that feels like a wonderful treat.

Serves 4

FOR THE ICE CREAM
8 very ripe bananas
4 tablespoons crunchy nut butter (peanut, almond and cashew are all great)
12 medjool dates, pitted and roughly chopped

FOR THE HAZELNUT BROWNIE BITES
80g roasted hazelnuts
200g medjool dates, pitted
2 tablespoons raw cacao powder

FOR THE CHOCOLATE SAUCE
50g raw cacao powder
6 tablespoons date syrup
2 tablespoons coconut oil
3 tablespoons coconut milk

TO SERVE
berries
toasted hazelnuts (optional)
coconut chips (optional)

Start with the ice cream. Peel the bananas, chop them into thin slices and place in the freezer for at least 4 hours.

Meanwhile, make the brownie bites. Place the hazelnuts into a food processor and blitz until they're crushed, then add the dates and cacao and blend until a sticky mix forms. Scrape the mix out, press it into a baking tray, cover and leave in the fridge until you need it.

Once you're ready for your sundaes, make the chocolate sauce. To do this, just melt the cacao powder, date syrup and coconut oil together, then whisk in the coconut milk. Set aside to cool.

Take the bananas out the freezer and let them defrost for a few minutes. Meanwhile, chop the brownie mix into bite-sized chunks.

Place the bananas into a food processor and blend for a minute or so, until totally smooth and resembling soft-serve ice cream. Now add the nut butter and blend for another few seconds. Stir in the dates (don't blend them in; you want them to be chunky).

Put a few brownie bites and berries at the bottom of 4 serving glasses or bowls, then add a scoop or 2 of ice cream, more brownie bites, chocolate sauce and toasted hazelnuts or coconut chips, if you like.

Serve straight away to stop the ice cream from melting!

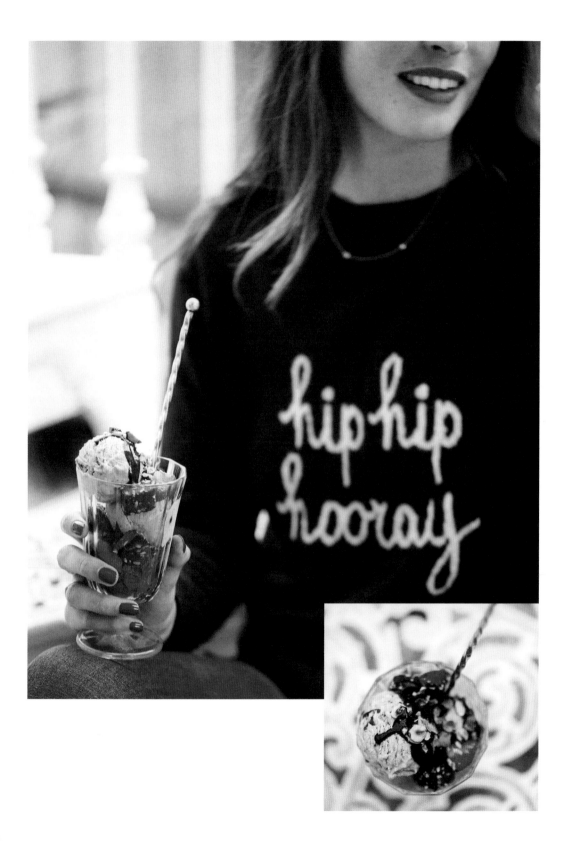

RECIPE INDEX

INDEX

THANK YOU

Every time I write a book I feel the list of people I want to thank gets longer and longer, as more incredible people enter my life and support Deliciously Ella!

It goes without saying that my readers get the biggest thank you. You've made my entire career possible and I'll forever be grateful for your daily support and enthusiasm for what I do, it inspires me so much and it's the reason that I continue to share recipes and ideas with the world. Together we've created a really special community, and I'm incredibly proud of the journey that we're sharing.

To my husband, Matthew, it's hard to find the right words to thank you for everything you do every day. The unending kindness and encouragement you show me is unbelievable: not only have you become my sounding board for every idea, you also help me nurture and grow the idea and inspire me to push myself in everything I do. You've motivated me to aim higher, believe in myself more and – most importantly – be the best and kindest person I can be, for which I am forever grateful.

Our team at Deliciously Ella and MaE Deli also deserve a huge thank you. Serena, Jess and Laura Kate are my daily support at Deliciously Ella and allow me to share more with you. I can't thank them enough for their hard work, laughter, creativity and positive energy, as well as their amazing ability to eat as much as I do and recipe test every day!

Our team at MaE are building an amazing company with Matthew and me, which allows us to share my philosophy with so many more people and that makes me so incredibly happy. Isabella, Tom, Dan, Alan, Holly, Betty, Ed and Lorna.... You're wonderful.

Thank you to Cathryn, Gordy, Siobhan, Chekka and everyone else at WME that supports Deliciously Ella. Your advice and guidance is invaluable and there's no way that I could have grown Deliciously Ella into what it is now without your encouragement and guidance.

Liz, Louise, Vickie and the team at Yellow Kite and Hodder, thank you all so much for believing in what I'm doing. It means the world to me to have such a dedicated publisher that shares my vision and really believes in the message I want to share with you all. Working together is always an incredibly collaborative, creative process and that really makes the book so special.

It's also thanks to Miranda, Clare, Rosie, Ellie, Polly and Lucy that the books look and feel so beautiful. Your hard work and imagination has brought my vision to life in a way that's so much better than I could have imagined. Thanks to you the recipes look stunning and I hope will inspire more people to get cooking! Thank you for helping me share this with the world in the best possible way.

The advice herein is not intended to replace the services of trained health professionals, or to be a substitute for medical advice. You are advised to consult with your health care professional with regard to matters relating to your health, and in particular regarding matters that may require diagnosis or medical attention.

First published in Great Britain in 2017 by Yellow Kite
An Imprint of Hodder & Stoughton
An Hachette UK company
1
Copyright © Ella Mills 2017
Photography © Clare Winfield 2016

The right of Ella Mills to be identified as the Author of the Work has been asserted by her in accordance with the Copyright, Designs and Patents Act 1988.

All rights reserved. No part of this publication may be reproduced, stored in the retrieval system, or transmitted, in any form or by any means without the prior written permission of the publisher, nor be otherwise circulated in any form of binding or cover other than that in which it is published and without a similar condition being imposed on the subsequent purchaser.

A CIP catalogue record for this title is available from the British Library.

Hardback ISBN: 978 1 473 61951 7
eBook ISBN: 978 1 473 61950 0

Publisher: Liz Gough
Design and Art Direction: Miranda Harvey
Photography: Clare Winfield
Editor: Lucy Bannell
Photo Shoot Co-ordinator: Ruth Ferrier
Index: Hilary Bird
Food Stylist: Rosie Reynolds
Cover Food stylist: Eleanor Mulligan
Assistant Food Stylists: Eleanor Mulligan, Adam Bush, Anna Hiddleston
Props Stylist: Polly Webb-Wilson
Cover Props Stylist: Cynthia Blackett
Make-up Artist: Laurey Simmons

Printed and bound in China by C&C Offset Printing Co Ltd.

Hodder & Stoughton policy is to use papers that are natural, renewable and recyclable products and made from wood grown in sustainable forests. The logging and manufacturing processes are expected to conform to the environmental regulations of the country of origin.

Yellow Kite
Hodder & Stoughton Ltd
Carmelite House
50 Victoria Embankment
London EC4 0DZ

www.yellowkitebooks.co.uk
www.hodder.co.uk

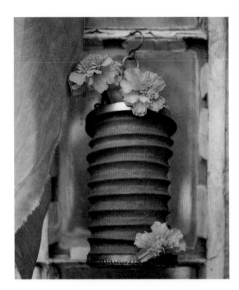